Milady's Standard Professional Barbering Exam Review

Maura Scali-Sheahan

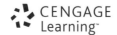
CENGAGE
Learning™

Australia   Canada   Mexico   Singapore   Spain   United Kingdom   United States

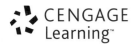

CENGAGE
Learning™

Milady's Standard
Professional Barbering Exam
Review
Maura
Scali-Sheahan

President, Milady:
Dawn Gerrain

Director of Editorial:
Sherry Gomoll

Acquisitions Editor:
Brad Hanson

Developmental Editor:
Jennifer Radalin

Editorial Assistant:
Jessica Burns

Director of Production:
Wendy A. Troeger

Production Editor:
Nina Tucciarelli

Director of Marketing:
Wendy Mapstone

Channel Manager:
Sandra Bruce

© 2008, 2006 Milady, a part of Cengage Learning

ALL RIGHTS RESERVED. No part of this work covered by the copyright herein may be reproduced, transmitted, stored or used in any form or by any means graphic, electronic, or mechanical, including but not limited to photocopying, recording, scanning, digitizing, taping, Web distribution, information networks, or information storage and retrieval systems, except as permitted under Section 107 or 108 of the 1976 United States Copyright Act, without the prior written permission of the publisher.

For product information and technology assistance, contact us at
Professional & Career Group Customer Support, 1-800-648-7450

For permission to use material from this text or product,
submit all requests online at **www.cengage.com/permissions**
Further permissions questions can be emailed to
permissionrequest@cengage.com

ExamView® and ExamView Pro® are registered trademarks of FSCreations, Inc. Windows is a registered trademark of the Microsoft Corporation used herein under license. Macintosh and Power Macintosh are registered trademarks of Apple Computer, Inc. Used herein under license.

Library of Congress Control Number: 2005016261

ISBN-13: 978-1-4018-7396-7

ISBN-10: 1-4018-7396-0

Cengage Learning
5 Maxwell Drive
Clifton Park, NY 12065-2919
USA

Cengage Learning products are represented in Canada by Nelson Education, Ltd.

For your lifelong learning solutions, visit
milady.cengage.com

Visit our corporate website at **www.cengage.com**

Notice to the Reader

Publisher does not warrant or guarantee any of the products described herein or perform any independent analysis in connection with any of the product information contained herein. Publisher does not assume, and expressly disclaims, any obligation to obtain and include information other than that provided to it by the manufacturer. The reader is expressly warned to consider and adopt all safety precautions that might be indicated by the activities described herein and to avoid all potential hazards. By following the instructions contained herein, the reader willingly assumes all risks in connection with such instructions. The publisher makes no representations or warranties of any kind, including but not limited to, the warranties of fitness for particular purpose or merchantability, nor are any such representations implied with respect to the material set forth herein, and the publisher takes no responsibility with respect to such material. The publisher shall not be liable for any special, consequential, or exemplary damages resulting, in whole or part, from the readers' use of, or reliance upon, this material.

Printed in Canada
6 7 11 10 09

Milady's Standard
Professional Barbering Exam Review

Contents iii

Foreword v

PART I: Chapter Review Tests 1

CHAPTER 1: Study Skills 1

CHAPTER 2: The History of Barbering 3

CHAPTER 3: Professional Image 6

CHAPTER 4: Bacteriology 11

CHAPTER 5: Infection Control and Safe Work Practices 16

CHAPTER 6: Implements, Tools, and Equipment 23

CHAPTER 7: Anatomy and Physiology 29

CHAPTER 8: Chemistry 38

CHAPTER 9: Electricity and Light Therapy 43

CHAPTER 10: Properties and Disorders of the Skin 47

CHAPTER 11: Properties and Disorders of the Hair and Scalp 56

CHAPTER 12: Treatment of the Hair and Scalp 66

CHAPTER 13: Men's Facial Massage and Treatments 75

CHAPTER 14: Shaving and Facial Hair Design 86

CHAPTER 15: Men's Haircutting and Styling 91

CHAPTER 16: Men's Hairpieces 102

CHAPTER 17: Women's Haircutting and Styling 106

CHAPTER 18: Chemical Texture Services 110

CHAPTER 19: Haircoloring and Lightening 121

CHAPTER 20: Nails and Manicuring 132

CHAPTER 21: Barbershop Management 136

CHAPTER 22: The Job Search 141

CHAPTER 23: State Board Preparation and Licensing Laws 143

PART II: Sample State Board Examinations **147**

Sample State Board Examination — Test 1 147

Sample State Board Examination — Test 2 163

Sample State Board Examination — Test 3 179

Answers to Chapter Review Tests 194

Answers to Sample State Board Examinations 206

PART III: Helpful Reminders for Examination Day **209**

Foreword

The purpose of this book is to assist barbering students in their preparation for state board examinations. The contents of this book mirror the changes and updates reflected in the 2005 revision of *Milady's Standard Professional Barbering* textbook and serves to provide examination candidates with an overall review of the material therein. This material review is presented in a multiple-choice test format, which represents the standard examination form adopted by the majority of state barber boards for written and computer-based examinations.

Part I, Chapter Review Tests, provides a comprehensive review test for each textbook chapter. These tests are designed to provide a detailed review of the subject matter found in each chapter and should be used by students to evaluate their personal level of understanding in a *specific* subject area. Students will then be able to identify subject areas in which they have a clear understanding and those areas that need additional review or study prior to completing the Sample State Board Examinations in Part II.

In Part II, three Sample State Board Examinations have been compiled from the chapter review tests. Each subject area is represented by several of the most universally relevant questions to that topic and its application to the field of barbering that *may* be included in a state board examination.

It is recommended that instructors review the questions in each 150-item test to determine the relevancy of the question topics to their particular state board exams. For example, some states may not require testing in nail histology or manicuring because the subject is not included in the barbering curriculum. Other states may not require testing in chemical services applications. Therefore it becomes the responsibility of barber instructors to provide students with *specific* guidance regarding the state board examination in their state.

Part III, Helpful Reminders for Examination Day, provides a general guideline for exam candidates to follow when preparing for written or computer-based and practical examinations. It is recommended that instructors review these guidelines as well, adapt the information to conform with the procedures of their state barber board, and share the results with their students.

PART I — Chapter Review Tests

DIRECTIONS: Read each statement carefully. Choose the word or phrase that most correctly completes the meaning of the statement and write the corresponding letter in the blank provided.

CHAPTER 1: STUDY SKILLS

1. The ability to learn and master new information is important to a student barber's success as a:
   a) barber   b) person
   c) student   d) barbershop owner   __C__

2. Personal study skills are tools that should help an individual:
   a) recall information   b) organize information
   c) store information   d) a, b, and c   _____

3. An individual's short-term memory may be improved through the use of:
   a) repetition   b) organization
   c) a and b   d) neither a nor b   _____

4. Acronyms, songs, rhymes, or any other devices that help an individual recall information are known as:
   a) organizers   b) mnemonics
   c) distracters   d) mind-maps   _____

5. Classifications that are used to identify the different ways in which people learn are called:
   a) learning tools   b) learning methods
   c) learning styles   d) learning stigmas   _____

6. The way in which an individual sees reality is the same as that individual's:
   a) preconception of reality   b) perception of reality
   c) prognosis of reality   d) purpose of reality   _____

7. For learning to take place, information and experiences must be:

   a) processed
   b) preconceived
   c) paralleled
   d) promulgated

   _____

8. An important aspect of developing effective study habits is to know:

   a) when to study
   b) where to study
   c) how to study
   d) a, b, and c

   _____

CHAPTER 2: THE HISTORY OF BARBERING

1. The word *barber* is derived from the Latin word *barba* meaning:
   a) to cut
   b) beard
   c) shave
   d) hairdresser

   b

2. The first culture to cultivate beauty in an extravagant fashion were the:
   a) Romans
   b) Africans
   c) Greeks
   d) Egyptians

   d

3. The barber Meryma'at is a historical figure of:
   a) Rome
   b) China
   c) Egypt
   d) Greece

   c

4. The use of braiding frequently denoted status within the tribes of:
   a) Israel
   b) Africa
   c) Mesopotamia
   d) Syria

   b

5. In 500 BC, barbering and hairstyling became highly developed arts in:
   a) Rome
   b) Africa
   c) Greece
   d) Egypt

   c

6. The man credited with the introduction of shaving and barbering services to Rome in 296 BC is:
   a) Caesar
   b) Meryma'at
   c) Alexander the Great
   d) Ticinius Mena

   d

7. In almost every early culture, an individual's hairstyle indicated:
   a) status
   b) personal style
   c) fashion
   d) age

   a

8. In ancient Rome, a woman's hair color indicated her:
   a) culture
   b) rank
   c) personal style
   d) age

   b

9. Throughout history, hair and beard trends were initiated by the:
   a) barbers of the country
   b) rulers of the country
   c) wealthy of the country
   d) upper classes of the country

   b

10. In early times, the beard was considered by almost all nations to be a sign of:
    a) peace   b) age
    c) status   d) wisdom

    c

11. During the Middle Ages, barbers practiced shaving, haircutting, and:
    a) medicine   b) business
    c) magic   d) astronomy

    a

12. Barber-surgeons participated in the practice of:
    a) bloodletting   b) teeth pulling
    c) surgery   d) a, b, and c

    d

13. The Latin word *tondere* means to:
    a) cut   b) shear
    c) trim   d) curl

    b

14. A shaved patch on the crown of the head is known as a:
    a) queue   b) tonsorial
    c) tonsure   d) fringe

    c

15. The symbol of the barber-surgeon evolved from the technical procedure of:
    a) pulling teeth   b) bloodletting
    c) suturing a wound   d) trimming beards

    b

16. The symbol of the barber-surgeons and modern-day barbers is the:
    a) barber razor   b) barber pole
    c) barber comb   d) barber sign

    b

17. By the nineteenth century, barbering was completely separated from religion and medicine and began to emerge as an independent:
    a) association   b) organization
    c) profession   d) guild

    c

18. During the late 1800s, the members of employer organizations were:
    a) journeymen barbers   b) student barbers
    c) master barbers   d) apprentice barbers

    c

19. In 1893, A. B. Moler established America's first barber:
    a) trade journal   b) association
    c) school   d) license

    c

4

20. America's first barber school was located in:
    a) Chicago   b) Boston
    c) St. Louis   d) St. Paul   *a*

21. The first state to pass a barber license law was:
    a) Minnesota   b) New York
    c) Illinois   d) Ohio   *a*

22. The purpose of the National Education Council was to establish the standardization of barber:
    a) poles   b) training
    c) licenses   d) uniforms   *b*

23. In 1929, the Associated Master Barbers of America adopted a Barber Code of Ethics to promote:
    a) barber schools   b) examinations
    c) professionalism   d) regulation   *c*

24. State barber boards are primarily interested in maintaining high standards of:
    a) appliances   b) tools
    c) products   d) competency   *d*

25. One key function of state barber boards is to protect the health, safety, and welfare of the:
    a) profession   b) barbers
    c) public   d) board members   *c*

CHAPTER 3: PROFESSIONAL IMAGE

1. Personality, personal hygiene, and attitude are all aspects of an individual's:
   a) grooming
   b) barbering skills
   c) professional image
   d) health
   _____

2. Prior learning and life experiences are also known as:
   a) destiny
   b) life skills
   c) study skills
   d) image
   _____

3. Values guide how we act; how we act is based on our beliefs and:
   a) what we think and feel
   b) what we feel
   c) what we see
   d) neither a, b, or c
   _____

4. Beliefs are attitudes that originate from an individual's:
   a) thoughts
   b) values
   c) desires
   d) ideas
   _____

5. Speech, appearance, behavior, and manners are all signs of an individual's:
   a) education
   b) aggressiveness
   c) vitality
   d) personality
   _____

6. The only difference between a good day and a bad day is an individual's:
   a) luck
   b) timing
   c) attitude
   d) purpose
   _____

7. The art of being tactful is known as:
   a) diplomacy
   b) indifference
   c) diplomatic immunity
   d) callousness
   _____

8. To be responsive to others' ideas, feelings, and opinions is known as:
   a) responsibility
   b) reception
   c) receptivity
   d) resonance
   _____

9. Hygiene is the science that deals with:
   a) disease transmittal
   b) healthful living
   c) health breakdown
   d) bacteriology
   _____

10. The primary purpose of practicing hygiene is to:
    a) control population growth
    b) promote disease
    c) wash daily
    d) preserve health
    _____

11. Personal hygiene deals with the health preservation of the:
    a) individual   b) community
    c) town   d) county   _____

12. Rest allows the body to recover from:
    a) relaxation   b) a night's sleep
    c) the day's activities   d) good nutrition   _____

13. Walking, dancing, and sports are all forms of:
    a) nutrition   b) rest
    c) exercise   d) good posture   _____

14. Improved blood circulation is a benefit of:
    a) personal hygiene   b) rest
    c) exercise   d) hygiene   _____

15. Good nutrition is one of the major factors necessary to preserve:
    a) good health   b) irritability
    c) general fatigue   d) poor health   _____

16. Practicing stress management helps an individual live a/an:
    a) nutritious life   b) active life
    c) wild and crazy life   d) healthy life   _____

17. The body operates as a unit with:
    a) nutrition   b) posture
    c) stress management   d) the mind   _____

18. The barber who practices correct posture will find that it helps to minimize:
    a) skin discoloration   b) body fatigue
    c) balance   d) muscular coordination   _____

19. For a comfortable sitting posture, keep the soles of the feet:
    a) on the floor   b) crossed
    c) extended   d) raised   _____

20. To avoid back strain while reading, writing, or studying, sit:
    a) toward the back of the chair   b) in a slouching position
    c) on the forward part of the chair   d) rigidly upright   _____

21. The study of human characteristics as applied to specific work environments is:
    a) isometrics   b) anatomy
    c) ergonomics   d) physiology   _____

22. The psychology of getting along well with others is known as:
   a) human emotions   b) human relations
   c) human understanding d) human characteristics   _____

23. One of the barber's most important human relations skills is the ability to:
   a) cut hair   b) communicate effectively
   c) talk excessively   d) be quiet   _____

24. Listening skills, voice, speech, and conversation skills are aspects of effective:
   a) emotions   b) personality
   c) mannerisms   d) communication   _____

25. Three steps that can be used to ascertain a client's service expectations are:
   a) ask, suggest,   b) organize thoughts,
      promote   show, suggest
   c) organize thoughts, d) tell, clarify, repeat   _____
      clarify, repeat

26. Proper behavior and business dealings with employers, clients, and coworkers is called:
   a) professional   b) professional ethics
      technique
   c) career guidance   d) behavioral characteristics _____

27. Proper ethical practices help to increase business and to build:
   a) opposition   b) competition
   c) confidence   d) disloyalty   _____

28. Proper conduct and behavior in the barbershop is the best method for building a:
   a) professional skill   b) student organization
   c) trade association   d) good reputation   _____

29. To become a successful professional barber, individuals should follow the rule of:
   a) questionable   b) good ethical practices
      business practices
   c) high-priced services d) arrogant attitude   _____

30. A basic principle that forms the foundation of success includes:
   a) visualization   b) respect others
   c) practice new   d) a, b, and c   _____
      behaviors

31. A desire for change creates:
    a) motivation   b) sympathy
    c) apathy   d) manipulation   _____

32. Extrinsic motivation may stem from:
    a) family   b) teachers
    c) friends   d) a, b, and c   _____

33. The most effective form of motivation is:
    a) extrinsic   b) intrinsic
    c) external   d) individual   _____

34. A well-thought-out process for long-term planning and success requires:
    a) self-deception   b) self-indulgence
    c) self-management   d) self-aggrandizement _____

35. Dreams and plans for the future are also known as:
    a) goals   b) rights
    c) expectations   d) wishes   _____

36. Important elements of goal setting include planning, reexamination, and:
    a) irritability   b) stubbornness
    c) flexibility to change d) shortsightedness _____

37. Effective time management techniques include:
    a) prioritizing and   b) scheduling and rewards
       problem solving
    c) a and b   d) neither a nor b   _____

38. Personal grooming is an extension of:
    a) personal hygiene   b) barbering
    c) sanitization   d) politeness   _____

39. It will be helpful to a barber's success to develop a:
    a) list of good stories b) apathetic attitude
    c) business-only attitude d) pleasing attitude _____

40. Thoughtfulness of others is considered to be the foundation of:
    a) good grooming   b) vigor
    c) vitality   d) politeness   _____

41. When suggesting additional products or services to clients, always be:
    a) tactful   b) pushy
    c) critical   d) judgmental   _____

42. Settle all disputes and differences to the satisfaction of the:
   - a) barber
   - b) shop employees
   - c) shop owner
   - d) client _____

43. The professional barber's best advertisement is his/her:
   - a) personal appearance
   - b) reputation for gossip
   - c) fast talking
   - d) persuasiveness _____

44. The successful barber avoids the use of:
   - a) safety standards
   - b) listening to clients
   - c) profane language
   - d) common sense _____

45. Unpleasant clients in the barbershop should be treated with:
   - a) sarcasm and contempt
   - b) profanity
   - c) disgust and impatience
   - d) patience and courtesy _____

46. In the presence of clients, the professional barber avoids:
   - a) courtesy
   - b) smoking
   - c) cooperation
   - d) tactfulness _____

47. Teaching and learning should not be interfered with by:
   - a) personal calls
   - b) good attendance
   - c) ethical training
   - d) safety rules _____

48. Accidents can be prevented or minimized if students carefully observe the:
   - a) school regulations
   - b) teacher's demonstrations
   - c) safety rules
   - d) license laws _____

49. Students are expected to comply with:
   - a) state barber board rules
   - b) barber school rules
   - c) safety rules
   - d) a, b, and c _____

50. The protection of the health, safety, and welfare of the public as it relates to barbering is the responsibility of:
   - a) state barber boards
   - b) barbering schools
   - c) barbers and barbering students
   - d) a, b, and c _____

CHAPTER 4: BACTERIOLOGY

1. Bacteriology is the scientific study of:
   a) chemicals   b) plants
   c) microorganisms   d) human tissues   c

2. Bacteria are microscopic, one-celled:
   a) microorganisms   b) plant forms
   c) animals   d) chemicals   a

3. Bacteria are most numerous:
   a) on a clean body   b) on clean implements
   c) in dirty places   d) on clean towels   c

4. Pathogenic bacteria produce:
   a) health   b) disease
   c) antitoxins   d) beneficial effects   b

5. Harmful bacteria are called:
   a) saprophyte bacteria   b) pathogenic bacteria
   c) nonpathogenic   d) protozoa bacteria   b
      bacteria

6. Bacteria live and grow best in:
   a) cold places   b) dry places
   c) dirty places   d) clean places   c

7. Bacteria are commonly known as:
   a) antiseptics   b) disinfectants
   c) germs or microbes d) saprophytes   c

8. Bacteria are visible only with the aid of:
   a) a microscope   b) tinted glasses
   c) eyeglasses   d) sunglasses   a

9. Cocci are bacteria that have a:
   a) round shape   b) rod shape
   c) corkscrew shape   d) curved shape   a

10. Bacilli are bacteria that have a:
    a) corkscrew shape   b) round shape
    c) rod shape   d) curved shape   c

11. Spirilla are bacteria that have a:
    a) round shape   b) corkscrew shape
    c) rod shape   d) flat shape   b

12. Pus-forming organisms that grow in clusters and cause abscesses, pustules, pimples, and boils are:
    a) streptococci bacteria   b) staphylococci bacteria
    c) diplococci bacteria   d) spirilla bacteria

    b

13. Pus-forming organisms that grow in chains and cause strep throat, tonsillitis, lung diseases, and blood poisoning are:
    a) streptococci bacteria   b) bacilli bacteria
    c) diplococci bacteria   d) spirilla bacteria

    a

14. Bacteria that grow in pairs, causing pneumonia and gonorrhea are:
    a) streptococci bacteria   b) staphylococci bacteria
    c) diplococci bacteria   d) spirilla bacteria

    c

15. Bacteria that produce diseases such as tetanus, influenza, typhoid fever, tuberculosis, and diphtheria are:
    a) streptococci bacteria   b) bacilli bacteria
    c) diplococci bacteria   d) spirilla bacteria

    b

16. The type of bacteria that causes syphilis and Lyme disease is:
    a) streptococci bacteria   b) bacilli bacteria
    c) diplococci bacteria   d) spirilla bacteria

    d

17. Pustules and boils contain:
    a) nonpathogenic organisms   b) pathogenic bacteria
    c) sweat   d) ringworm

    b

18. Hairlike projections that propel bacteria through liquids are called:
    a) motile   b) mobile
    c) flagella or cilia   d) hair shafts

    c

19. The active stage of bacteria is also known as the:
    a) spore-forming stage   b) vegetative stage
    c) inactive stage   d) dormant stage

    b

20. The inactive stage of bacteria is also known as the:
    a) spore-forming stage   b) vegetative stage
    c) active stage   d) reproductive stage

    a

21. During the active stage, bacteria:
    a) vegetate   b) lie dormant
    c) grow and reproduce   d) form spores

    c

22. During the inactive stage, bacteria:
    - a) die
    - b) lie dormant
    - c) grow
    - d) reproduce

    b

23. Bacteria reproduce by dividing in:
    - a) half
    - b) quarters
    - c) sixths
    - d) eighths

    a

24. The process of cell division is known as:
    - a) halitosis
    - b) bromhidrosis
    - c) mitosis
    - d) anhidrosis

    c

25. Toxin means:
    - a) deodorant
    - b) poison
    - c) styptic
    - d) fumigant

    b

26. The presence of pus is a sign of:
    - a) infection
    - b) impurities
    - c) immunity
    - d) healing

    a

27. A boil is an example of a:
    - a) general infection
    - b) local infection
    - c) nonpathogenic bacteria
    - d) contagious disease

    b

28. An example of a general infection is:
    - a) a boil
    - b) blood poisoning
    - c) nose discharge
    - d) a skin lesion

    b

29. A communicable disease is:
    - a) not transmittable
    - b) usually a local infection
    - c) transmitted from person to person
    - d) caused by nonpathogenic bacteria

    c

30. A contagious disease that will prevent a barber from servicing clients is:
    - a) tuberculosis
    - b) viral infections
    - c) the common cold
    - d) a, b, or c

    d

31. Disease may be spread by:
    - a) disinfectants
    - b) soiled hands
    - c) antiseptics
    - d) sanitized implements

    b

32. Bacteria can enter the body through:
    - a) a healthy scalp
    - b) unbroken skin
    - c) broken skin
    - d) oily skin

    c

33. Resistance to disease is known as:
    a) infection   b) immunity
    c) parasite   d) fungus   *b*

34. Disease-producing organisms that live only by
    penetrating cells and becoming a part of them are:
    a) viruses   b) germs
    c) bacteria   d) microbes   *a*

35. Organisms that can live on their own are:
    a) plasmas   b) viruses
    c) bacteria   d) parasites   *c*

36. Disease-producing bacteria or viruses that are carried
    through the body in blood or body fluids are known as:
    a) bloodborne   b) bloodborne nonpathogens
       parasites
    c) bloodborne   d) bloodborne disorders   *c*
       pathogens

37. Poisoning due to pathogenic bacteria is called:
    a) styptic   b) sepsis
    c) asepsis   d) spirilla   *b*

38. An absence of disease germs is known as:
    a) toxin   b) sepsis
    c) poisoned   d) asepsis   *d*

39. Symptoms such as itching, burning, or pain
    are called:
    a) objective symptoms   b) subjective symptoms   *b*
    c) parasitic symptoms   d) internal symptoms

40. Plant or animal organisms that live on another
    living organism without giving anything in return
    are called:
    a) parasites   b) saprophytes   *a*
    c) bacteria   d) appendages

41. Ringworm is caused by a/an:
    a) animal parasite   b) poison ivy
    c) bacterial parasite   d) plant parasite   *d*

42. Pediculosis is caused by:
    a) the itch mite   b) the body or head louse   *b*
    c) scabies   d) ringworm

14

43. There is no vaccine for the:
    a) Hepatitis virus   b) Hepatitis A virus
    c) Hepatitis B virus   d) Hepatitis C virus   _d_

44. AIDS stands for:
    a) acquired infection   b) actualized immune
       deficiency syndrome   deficit symptom
    c) acquired immuno-   d) actualized infection   _C_
       deficiency syndrome   deficiency syndrome

45. The virus that causes AIDS is:
    a) HIB   b) HIV
    c) ARC   d) STD   _b_

46. Once HIV has entered the bloodstream, the production
    of antibodies is called:
    a) retrovirus   b) anabolism
    c) seroconversion   d) arrhythmia   _C_

47. One of the most common methods of transmitting the
    AIDS virus is:
    a) by kissing an infected b) by shaking hands with
       person   an infected person
    c) through the air   d) through sexual contact   _d_
                                 with an infected person

48. The most likely manner in which HIV may be transmitted
    in the barbershop is by:
    a) shaking hands with   b) blood-to-blood contact
       an infected person
    c) using a soiled   d) using a sanitized comb with   _b_
       headrest   an infected person

49. A person can be infected with HIV without having
    symptoms for up to:
    a) 1 year   b) 20 years
    c) 11 years   d) 50 years   _C_

50. The symptom stages of AIDS appear in the following order:
    a) HIV, ARC, AIDS   b) STD, AIDS, ARC
    c) STD, HIV, AIDS   d) HIV, STD, ARC   _a_

CHAPTER 5: INFECTION CONTROL AND SAFE WORK PRACTICES

1. Bacteria, viruses, and fungi in the barbershop act as:
   a) decontaminants
   b) immunity producers
   c) contaminants
   d) sanitizers _____

2. The removal of pathogens from tools and surfaces is known as:
   a) decontamination
   b) contamination
   c) sepsis
   d) cleaning _____

3. The process of decontamination may be achieved through:
   a) sterilization
   b) sanitation
   c) disinfection
   d) a, b, and c _____

4. State barber boards and health departments require only:
   a) sterilization procedures
   b) sanitation procedures
   c) disinfection procedures
   d) disinfection and sanitation procedures _____

5. The highest level of decontamination is:
   a) sterilization
   b) soap and water
   c) disinfection
   d) sanitation _____

6. The process of thoroughly cleaning a tool or surface to its optimum level of decontamination in the barbershop is known as:
   a) sterilization
   b) sanitizer
   c) disinfectant
   d) disinfection or sanitation _____

7. Sanitation is the process of:
   a) keeping bacteria alive
   b) destroying only beneficial microorganisms
   c) destroying offensive odors
   d) keeping objects clean and sanitary _____

8. Chemical agents that are used to destroy most bacteria and some viruses are:
   a) antiseptics
   b) disinfectants
   c) toners
   d) alcohols _____

9. The most effective sanitizing agents used to destroy pathogenic bacteria are:
   a) antiseptics
   b) astringents
   c) chemical disinfectants
   d) solutions _____

10. A disinfectant that contains the properties of a bactericide, fungicide, pseudomonacide, virucide, and tuberculocide is considered to be a/an:
   a) minimal disinfectant   b) hospital-level disinfectant
   c) deodorizer   d) antiseptic   _____

11. Antiseptics are primarily used on:
   a) the skin   b) cutting implements
   c) dirty floors   d) brushes and combs   _____

12. An example of an antiseptic is:
   a) bleach   b) chlorine
   c) hydrogen peroxide   d) 99% isopropyl alcohol   _____

13. The sanitizing agent that sodium hypochlorite contains is:
   a) quats   b) alcohol
   c) chlorine   d) sulfonated oil   _____

14. An example of moist-heat sanitizing is:
   a) baking in an oven   b) fumigation
   c) boiling water   d) disinfection   _____

15. The sanitizing agents most often used in barbershops are:
   a) boiling water   b) baking in ovens
   c) chemical disinfectants d) steam pressure sanitizers   _____

16. Quaternary ammonium compounds (quats) are commonly used:
   a) disinfectants   b) styptics
   c) fumigants   d) deodorants   _____

17. For effective sanitization, the minimum strength of a quat solution used to sanitize implements is:
   a) 10%   b) 1:2000
   c) 1:1000   d) 20%   _____

18. Sharp metallic implements may be sanitized with:
   a) kerosene   b) styptic
   c) a disinfectant   d) hydrogen peroxide   _____

19. The function of commercially prepared products for use on clippers is to:
   a) cool   b) lubricate
   c) disinfect   d) a, b, and/or c   _____

20. To prepare a 1:1000 quat solution, the barber needs to mix:
    a) 1¼ ounces quat to one gallon of water
    b) 1 ounce quat to one gallon of water
    c) 1½ ounces quat to two gallons of water
    d) 1¼ ounces quat to two gallons of water _____

21. When a solute is dissolved in a solvent, the result is a:
    a) secretion
    b) solution
    c) sebum
    d) solvency _____

22. In a 10% solution of sodium hypochlorite, the percentage of water is:
    a) 10%
    b) 50%
    c) 90%
    d) 100% _____

23. A covered receptacle containing a disinfectant solution is called a/an:
    a) dry sanitizer
    b) cabinet sanitizer
    c) wet sanitizer
    d) oven sanitizer _____

24. A wet sanitizer should contain:
    a) a disinfectant solution
    b) 30% alcohol
    c) an antiseptic solution
    d) 2% formalin _____

25. Electric sanitizers that use lamps or bulbs to keep sanitized tools sanitary are:
    a) infrared cabinets
    b) ultraviolet-ray cabinets
    c) dry sanitizers
    d) light spectrum sanitizers _____

26. A dry sanitizer is most effective when it:
    a) has an open door
    b) contains an active fumigant
    c) contains hot steam
    d) contains an antiseptic _____

27. Before sanitizing any implement, it should be:
    a) wiped with a towel
    b) wiped with a tissue
    c) rinsed with water
    d) cleaned with soap and warm water _____

28. Phenols are used to:
    a) sanitize implements
    b) mix with disinfectants
    c) take the place of soap
    d) strengthen shampoos _____

29. The minimum effective disinfection strength of ethyl alcohol is:
    a) 60%
    b) 70%
    c) 80%
    d) 90% _____

30. The minimum effective disinfection strength of isopropyl alcohol is:
    a) 50%   b) 75%
    c) 88%   d) 99%   _____

31. The first step to using a chemical solution is to:
    a) measure the product   b) put on gloves
    c) read the directions   d) wear a lab coat or apron   _____

32. Chemicals used in a barbershop should be:
    a) kept in an unlocked   b) kept in open jars and bottles
       cabinet
    c) properly labeled   d) stored in a warm place   _____

33. Electrodes may be sanitized with:
    a) glycerin   b) disinfectant
    c) boiling water   d) boric acid   _____

34. Combs and brushes are best sanitized by immersion in a:
    a) deodorant solution   b) boric acid solution
    c) disinfectant solution d) glycerin solution   _____

35. For effective disinfection, a quat solution requires:
    a) a long contact time   b) a high strength
    c) a short contact time d) mixing with soap   _____

36. An example of a chemical agent used in sanitization is:
    a) boiling water   b) steam under pressure
    c) ultraviolet rays d) quats   _____

37. The Occupational Safety and Health Administration (OSHA) regulates and enforces safety and health in the workplace by:
    a) setting safety   b) selling safe products
       standards
    c) causing worker injury d) importing products   _____

38. Product descriptions and important data including content, associated hazards, combustion levels, and storage requirements are provided by:
    a) shop owners   b) barbers
    c) Material Safety   d) importers
       Data Sheets   _____

39. The responsibility of product safety rests with the:
    a) Food and   b) Occupational Safety and
       Drug Administration   Health Administration
    c) manufacturer   d) distributor   _____

40. The Right-to-Know Law requires that a notice be posted in work environments where:
   - a) break times are required
   - b) chemicals are used
   - c) nontoxic materials are used
   - d) toxic substances are present _____

41. A "professional" product is a product:
   - a) used by barbers
   - b) created by barbers
   - c) sold only to industry professionals
   - d) available over-the-counter by a retailer _____

42. A bulge in a plastic container most likely indicates:
   - a) poor packaging
   - b) an inferior plastic container
   - c) that contents are under pressure
   - d) a bubble in the plastic _____

43. Keep clean towels:
   - a) near dirty towels
   - b) in a clean, open cabinet
   - c) in a clean, closed cabinet
   - d) on a nearby shelf _____

44. Sanitized implements are best stored:
   - a) in a drawer
   - b) in an open cabinet
   - c) in a clean, closed container
   - d) on a shelf _____

45. Barbers should wash their hands:
   - a) in the morning
   - b) when they get dirty
   - c) morning and afternoon
   - d) before and after serving each client _____

46. Implements must be cleaned prior to immersion in a disinfectant solution to:
   - a) avoid solution contamination
   - b) comply with state board rules
   - c) comply with sanitation procedures
   - d) a, b, and c _____

47. A 6% hydrogen peroxide solution may be used as a/an:
   - a) eye wash
   - b) antiseptic
   - c) mouth wash
   - d) disinfectant _____

48. To be effective, the contact time needed for 99% isopropyl alcohol, 70% ethyl alcohol, and 10% sodium hypochlorite is:
   - a) 1 minute
   - b) 5 minutes
   - c) 10 minutes
   - d) 15 minutes _____

49. When a blood spill occurs, employ:
    a) a doctor
    b) disinfection
    c) universal precautions
    d) decontamination _____

50. A freshly laundered towel should be used:
    a) for every two clients
    b) for each client
    c) until it gets soiled
    d) over and over again _____

51. Headrest covers must be changed:
    a) for each client
    b) whenever they get soiled
    c) for every three
       clients
    d) for every other client _____

52. For sanitary reasons, combs should never be placed in:
    a) a dry sanitizer
    b) sealed envelopes
    c) uniform pockets
    d) dustproof cabinets _____

53. Objects dropped on the floor should not be used again until:
    a) washed with
       warm water
    b) wiped with a tissue
    c) sanitized
    d) wiped with a towel _____

54. Cream should be removed from jars with:
    a) the end of a
       used towel
    b) tips of fingers
    c) a clean spatula
    d) a comedone extractor _____

55. Hair or other waste materials on the floor of a barbershop should be:
    a) swept into a corner
    b) placed into a closed container
    c) hidden from view
    d) swept up at the end of
       the day _____

56. The alert and conscientious barber ensures client safety by using common sense and:
    a) products
    b) safety precautions
    c) trimmers
    d) record cards _____

57. When a serious accident occurs in the barbershop, call a/an:
    a) physician or 911
    b) other employee
    c) pharmacist
    d) telephone company _____

58. Most cuts or abrasions received in the barbershop are considered to be:
    a) minor wounds
    b) life-threatening
    c) the barber's fault
    d) trivial _____

59. Small nicks or cuts should be cleansed and treated with:
     a) an adhesive bandage b) soap and water
     c) styptic powder   d) styptic pencil   _____

60. Client emergency contact information should be
     maintained on the:
     a) appointment book   b) barber's station
     c) client record card   d) client list   _____

CHAPTER 6: IMPLEMENTS, TOOLS, AND EQUIPMENT

1. The most desirable type of hair comb is made of:
   a) plastic   b) metal
   c) bone   d) hard rubber   _____

2. To keep rubber combs in good condition, avoid contact with:
   a) dry air   b) cool air
   c) heat   d) metallic implements   _____

3. The French type of haircutting shears:
   a) has no finger brace   b) has one finger brace
   c) has two finger braces d) does not have a shank   _____

4. Shears with fine cutting edges can be poor cutting tools if they are:
   a) not set correctly   b) oiled
   c) sanitized with alcohol d) sharpened   _____

5. When holding haircutting shears properly, the barber places the thumb in the thumb grip of the:
   a) shank   b) still blade
   c) moving blade   d) finger grip   _____

6. While combing through the hair during a haircut service, the shears should be:
   a) resting on the   b) closed and resting in
      counter top   the barber's palm
   c) in the barber's   d) held in the hand that is not
      pocket   holding the comb   _____

7. The two main types of shear grinds are plain:
   a) thinning   b) notched
   c) corrugated   d) texturizing   _____

8. Clippers with a single cutting head usually have:
   a) a lever on the   b) low performance
      side of the unit
   c) detachable blades   d) plastic blades   _____

9. Electric clippers are driven by rotary motor, magnetic motor, or:
   a) circular motor   b) pivot motor
   c) vibratory motor   d) motor action   _____

10. Rotary motor clippers use:
    a) guards   b) a power screw adjustment
    c) detachable blades   d) many moving parts   _____

11. Pivot motor clippers have a/an:
    a) blade-adjusting   b) low performance
    lever
    c) detachable blades   d) plastic blades   _____

12. The type of motor clippers that operate by means of an
    alternating spring and magnetic mechanism are:
    a) all electric clippers   b) pivot motor clippers
    c) vibratory motor   d) rotary motor clippers   _____
    clippers

13. When haircutting, most detail and fine finish work is
    performed with the electric:
    a) rotary motor clipper   b) trimmer or outliner
    c) pivot motor clipper   d) shear   _____

14. Clipper blades are usually made of:
    a) tempered nickel   b) chrome
    c) hard rubber   d) carbon steel   _____

15. Clipper guards are also known as:
    a) detachable blades   b) safety guards
    c) attachment combs   d) clip-ons   _____

16. The clipper blade size that leaves the hair the longest is:
    a) size 1   b) size 2
    c) size $1\frac{1}{2}$ d) size 3   _____

17. The size clipper blade that produces the shortest cut is:
    a) size 0   b) size 0000
    c) size 000   d) size 00   _____

18. The first step in sanitizing clippers and trimmers is to:
    a) brush off hair   b) immerse blades in blade wash
    particles
    c) immerse blades   d) spray with disinfectant _____
    in water

19. The main consideration in the purchase of a straight
    razor is the:
    a) handle design   b) color
    c) weight   d) quality   _____

20. A straight razor is properly balanced when:
    a) the weight of the   b) the weight of the blade equals
       head equals that   that of the handle
       of the tang
    c) the weight of the   d) it does not pivot   _____
       blade does not equal
       that of the handle

21. The two types of razors are the conventional straight
    razor and the:
    a) cut-throat razor   b) stropping razor
    c) changeable-   d) steel razor   _____
       blade razor

22. The grind of a razor refers to the shape of the:
    a) tang   b) heel
    c) blade   d) handle   _____

23. The size of a razor is measured by the blade's:
    a) length   b) thickness
    c) sharpness   d) length and width   _____

24. The razor finish that lasts the longest is the:
    a) polished steel finish   b) chromium plated finish
    c) nickel plated finish   d) silver plated finish   _____

25. The temper of a razor indicates its degree of:
    a) heat   b) hardness
    c) cutting edge   d) balance   _____

26. A crocus finish on the blade of a razor is also known as:
    a) nickel plated finish   b) silver plated finish
    c) plain steel finish   d) polished steel finish   _____

27. The width of the razor is measured in eighth inches or:
    a) quarter inches   b) half inches
    c) sixteenth inches   d) full inches   _____

28. Honing and stropping are necessary for such implements
    as:
    a) haircutting shears   b) thinning shears
    c) conventional straight   d) hair clippers   _____
       razors

29. A hone is made of:
    a) leather   b) abrasive material
    c) soap   d) canvas   _____

30. The purpose of a hone is to:
   a) grind the razor's edge b) smooth the razor's edge
   c) polish the razor's edge d) align the razor's cutting
                              teeth   _____

31. An example of a slow-cutting hone is the:
   a) steel hone   b) water hone
   c) Swaty hone   d) synthetic hone   _____

32. An example of a fast-cutting hone is the:
   a) water hone   b) Belgian hone
   c) synthetic hone   d) natural hone   _____

33. The position of the hone when being used should be:
   a) any position   b) perfectly flat
   c) upside down   d) on a slant   _____

34. The type of stroke to use when honing a razor is a/an:
   a) smooth and   b) herky-jerky
      even stroke
   c) irregular stroke   d) any kind of stroke   _____

35. When properly honed, the razor edge should be:
   a) blunt   b) coarse
   c) keen   d) rough   _____

36. Additional finishing on a leather strop is required when
   the razor edge is:
   a) keen   b) blunt
   c) sharp   d) coarse   _____

37. The purpose of a strop is to:
   a) grind the razor's edge b) smooth the razor's edge
   c) polish the razor's edge d) impart a cutting edge to
                              the razor   _____

38. Avoid strops made of:
   a) natural leather   b) imitation leather
   c) cowhide   d) horsehide   _____

39. The Russian strop is made of:
   a) horsehide   b) imitation leather
   c) cowhide   d) synthetic materials   _____

40. The shell or Russian shell strop is created from:
   a) cowhide   b) the rump area of the horse
   c) synthetic materials   d) canvas   _____

41. The direction used in razor stropping is:
    a) the same as that used in honing
    b) in a counterclockwise direction
    c) the reverse of that used in honing
    d) in a clockwise direction _____

42. When testing a honed razor edge, a disagreeable sound indicates that the cutting edge is:
    a) coarse
    b) keen
    c) blunt
    d) dull _____

43. The purpose of strop dressing is to:
    a) clean the strop leather
    b) improve draw and sharpening
    c) preserves the strop finish
    d) a, b, and c _____

44. Electric latherizers use:
    a) bar soap
    b) liquid cream soap
    c) soft soap
    d) powdered soap _____

45. The appliance designed for drying and styling hair in a single operation is the:
    a) diffuser
    b) hood dryer
    c) blow-dryer
    d) hair vacuum _____

46. The least acceptable method of removing loose hair after a haircut is the:
    a) small electric vacuum
    b) neck duster
    c) clean towel, properly folded
    d) paper neck strip _____

47. Conventional thermal irons and pressing combs are heated by:
    a) gas stoves
    b) electric stoves
    c) electric current
    d) infrared lamps _____

48. The appliance that is used to introduce water-soluble products into the skin is the:
    a) galvanic machine
    b) high-frequency machine
    c) tesla current
    d) stove _____

49. An implement used to press out blackheads is a/an:
    a) tweezers
    b) comedone extractor
    c) electric hair vacuum
    d) electric latherizer _____

50. The agency that a barber may call to determine whether straight razors, lather brushes, or neck dusters may be used in the barbershop is the:
    a) state health department
    b) state barber association
    c) state barber board
    d) state department of labor _____

CHAPTER 7: ANATOMY AND PHYSIOLOGY

1. A basic knowledge of anatomy and physiology assists
   barbers in analyzing and performing:
   a) first aid   b) shop ownership
   c) professional services   d) sanitation procedures   _____

2. The study of an organism's shape, structure, and the
   relationship of one body part to another is known as:
   a) anatomy   b) histology
   c) physiology   d) gross anatomy   _____

3. The study of an organism's observable structures as seen
   with the naked eye is:
   a) anatomy   b) histology
   c) physiology   d) gross anatomy   _____

4. The study of an organism's minute structures such as
   tissues and organs is called:
   a) anatomy   b) histology
   c) physiology   d) gross anatomy   _____

5. The study of an organism's functions, activities, and
   coordination of each body part is known as:
   a) anatomy   b) histology
   c) physiology   d) gross anatomy   _____

6. The basic units of the structure and function of all living
   things are:
   a) nuclei   b) cells
   c) centrosome   d) living matter   _____

7. Cells contain a colorless jellylike substance called:
   a) protoplasm   b) protein
   c) fat   d) mineral   _____

8. Food materials for cellular growth and self-repair are
   found in the:
   a) nucleus   b) membrane
   c) cytoplasm   d) centrosome   _____

9. The nucleus of the cell controls its activity and
   facilitates:
   a) cell division   b) self-repair
   c) food production   d) reproduction   _____

10. Cells of the human body reproduce through:
    a) direct division   b) amitosis
    c) indirect division d) anabolism   _____

11. A series of changes occurs in the nucleus of a human cell before it divides into:
    a) four cells   b) two cells
    c) three cells   d) five cells   _____

12. Metabolism consists of two phases, anabolism and:
    a) mitosis   b) cataphoresis
    c) amitosis   d) catabolism   _____

13. Body cells absorb water, food, and oxygen during:
    a) anabolism   b) catabolism
    c) mitosis   d) amitosis   _____

14. The energy needed for muscular effort is released during:
    a) mitosis   b) amitosis
    c) anabolism   d) catabolism   _____

15. Groups of cells that are similar in shape, size, structure, and function are:
    a) muscles   b) tissues
    c) organs   d) systems   _____

16. Organs generally consist of two or more different:
    a) systems   b) muscles
    c) tissues   d) cells   _____

17. Groups of organs that act together to perform one or more functions are:
    a) muscles   b) systems
    c) tissues   d) organelles   _____

18. The heart is an example of a/an:
    a) system   b) tissue
    c) cell   d) organ   _____

19. The human body consists of:
    a) five systems   b) seven systems
    c) ten systems   d) fifteen systems   _____

20. The skeletal system is important because it:
    a) covers the body   b) supplies blood to the body
    c) shapes and supports d) carries nerve messages   _____
       the body

21. The skull consists of eight cranial bones and:
    a) eight facial bones b) ten facial bones
    c) twelve facial bones d) fourteen facial bones   _____

22. The skull is the:
    a) bone of the arm   b) skeleton of the head
    c) facial nerve of   d) bone of the neck   _____
       the head

23. The occipital bone forms the back and base of the:
    a) neck   b) cranium
    c) upper jaw   d) forehead   _____

24. The parietal bones form the top and sides of the:
    a) face   b) cranium
    c) cheeks   d) neck   _____

25. The frontal bone forms the:
    a) upper jaw   b) lower jaw
    c) forehead   d) cheek   _____

26. The temporal bones form the:
    a) forehead   b) lower jaw
    c) Adam's apple   d) sides of the head   _____

27. The cervical vertebrae form the upper part of the spinal
    column at the:
    a) back of the neck   b) front of the neck
    c) side of the neck   d) front of the skull   _____

28. The sphenoid bone joins together all the bones of the:
    a) nose   b) cranium
    c) ear   d) neck   _____

29. The nasal bones form the:
    a) tip of the nose   b) back of the nose
    c) bridge of the nose   d) inner walls of the nose   _____

30. The zygomatic or malar bones form the:
    a) outer walls   b) mouth
       of the nose
    c) cheeks   d) U-shaped bone in throat   _____

31. Maxillae are bones that form the:
    a) lower jaw   b) upper jaw
    c) eye socket   d) forehead   _____

32. The mandible bone forms the:
    a) upper jaw   b) lower jaw
    c) cheek   d) nose   _____

33. The technical name for the "Adam's apple" is the:
    a) chin bone   b) cheek bone
    c) hyoid bone   d) jaw bone   _____

34. The muscular system covers, shapes, and supports the:
    a) skeletal system   b) nervous system
    c) circulatory system   d) digestive system   _____

35. One of the functions of the muscular system is to:
    a) circulate the blood   b) nourish the body
    c) produce body   d) produce marrow   _____
       movements

36. Activities of the muscular system are dependent on the
    skeletal system and the:
    a) lymphatic system   b) digestive system
    c) nervous system   d) circulatory system   _____

37. The more fixed attachment of a muscle to the bone is
    called the:
    a) origin   b) insertion
    c) joint   d) ligament   _____

38. The more movable attachment of a muscle to the bone
    is called the:
    a) insertion   b) origin
    c) belly   d) aponeurosis   _____

39. Muscles controlled by the will are known as:
    a) involuntary muscles   b) voluntary muscles
    c) cardiac muscles   d) nonstriated muscles   _____

40. Muscles not controlled by the will are called:
    a) skeletal muscles   b) voluntary muscles
    c) involuntary muscles   d) striated muscles   _____

41. Muscle tissue may be stimulated by massage, electric
    current, and:
    a) heat and light rays   b) nerve impulses and
                                        chemicals
    c) moist heat   d) a, b, and c   _____

42. Muscles of the scalp include the epicranius, frontalis,
    occipitalis, and the:
    a) aponeurosis   b) orbicularis oculi
    c) procerus   d) corrugator   _____

43. The muscle that produces vertical lines and causes
    frowning is the:
    a) buccinator   b) corrugator
    c) procerus   d) aponeurosis   _____

44. The procerus is associated with the:
    a) mouth   b) nose
    c) ears   d) eyes   _____

45. The levator labii superioris, depressor labii inferioris,
    levator anguli oris, and buccinator are associated with
    the:
    a) nose   b) eyes
    c) mouth   d) ears   _____

46. The orbicularis oris, mentalis, and zygomaticus relate to
    the:
    a) nose   b) lips
    c) eyes   d) forehead   _____

47. The corners of the mouth are drawn down by the:
    a) mentalis   b) triangularis
    c) risorius   d) zygomaticus   _____

48. Three auricularis muscles are associated with the:
    a) neck   b) eyes
    c) mouth   d) ears   _____

49. The platysma, sternocleidomastoideus, and trapezius are
    muscles related to the:
    a) mouth   b) nose   .
    c) neck   d) eyes   _____

50. The nervous system controls and coordinates all body:
    a) structures   b) functions
    c) cells   d) tissues   _____

51. The nervous system is composed of the brain, spinal
    cord, and their:
    a) blood vessels   b) nerves
    c) lymphatics   d) glands   _____

52. The main subdivisions of the nervous system are the
    cerebrospinal, peripheral, and:
    a) autonomic system   b) muscular system
    c) skeletal system   d) circulatory system   _____

53. Nerves are long, white cords made up of fibers from the:
    a) nerve cells   b) muscle cells
    c) bone cells   d) blood cells   _____

54. The largest and most complex nerve tissue in the body is/are the:
    a) lungs   b) spleen
    c) heart   d) brain   _____

55. The sensory nerves carry messages from the:
    a) brain to the muscles   b) sense organs to the brain
    c) brain to the   d) brain to the bones   _____
        spinal cord

56. The motor nerves carry nerve impulses from the:
    a) sense organs to   b) brain to the muscles
        the brain
    c) muscles to the brain   d) skin to the brain   _____

57. Nerves originate in the brain and the:
    a) lymphatic system   b) ganglia system
    c) spinal cord   d) cranium   _____

58. The cerebrospinal nervous system controls the:
    a) stomach muscles   b) heart muscles
    c) involuntary functions   d) voluntary functions and
                                   muscles   _____

59. Twelve pairs of cranial nerves branch out from the brain and reach parts of the:
    a) arms and hands   b) legs and feet
    c) abdomen and back   d) head, face, and neck   _____

60. The autonomic or sympathetic nervous system controls:
    a) voluntary muscles   b) mouth muscles
    c) involuntary muscles   d) hair color   _____
        and functions

61. The fifth cranial nerve, also known as the trifacial or trigeminal nerve, is the:
    a) chief sensory nerve   b) motor nerve that controls
        of the face   chewing
    c) neither a nor b   d) a and b   _____

62. The facial nerve that controls all the muscles used for facial expression is the:
    a) fifth cranial nerve   b) seventh cranial nerve
    c) eleventh cranial nerve   d) cervical nerve   _____

63. The spinal nerve branch that affects the muscles of the neck and back is the:
    a) fifth cranial nerve   b) seventh cranial nerve
    c) cervical nerve   d) eleventh cranial nerve   _____

64. Nerves may be stimulated by high-frequency current, moist heat, and:
    a) chemicals   b) light and heat rays
    c) massage   d) a, b, and c   _____

65. The nerve that supplies muscles and scalp at the back of the head and neck is the:
    a) fifth cranial nerve   b) seventh cranial nerve
    c) eleventh cranial nerve d) cervical nerve   _____

66. The cardiovascular or vascular system is also known as the:
    a) nervous system   b) lymphatic system
    c) circulatory system   d) blood-vascular system   _____

67. The blood-vascular system comprises the heart, arteries, veins, and:
    a) capillaries   b) lacteals
    c) duct glands   d) nodes   _____

68. The backflow of blood in the veins is prevented by:
    a) valves   b) vessels
    c) vesicles   d) verruca   _____

69. The upper heart chambers are called:
    a) ventricles   b) atria
    c) valves   d) pericardia   _____

70. The lower heart chambers are called:
    a) ventricles   b) arteries
    c) valves   d) atria   _____

71. Vessels that carry blood away from the heart are called:
    a) veins   b) capillaries
    c) arteries   d) lymphatics   _____

72. Vessels that carry blood back to the heart are:
    a) veins   b) capillaries
    c) arteries   d) lacteals   _____

73. Body cells receive food and eliminate waste products through the walls of the:
    a) veins   b) arteries
    c) capillaries   d) lacteals   _____

74. The two systems that control blood circulation are general circulation and:
    a) venous circulation   b) pulmonary circulation
    c) arterial circulation   d) capillary circulation   _____

75. The fluid part of the blood is called:
    a) plasma   b) platysma
    c) red blood cells   d) white blood cells   _____

76. Blood cells that carry oxygen to the body cells are the:
    a) white blood cells   b) blood platelets
    c) red blood cells   d) hemoglobin   _____

77. Blood cells that fight disease-causing germs are called:
    a) platelets   b) white blood cells
    c) red blood cells   d) plasma   _____

78. Those parts of the body not reached by the blood are nourished by:
    a) sweat   b) sebum
    c) juices   d) lymph   _____

79. The main sources of blood to the head, face, and neck are supplied by the
    a) jugular veins   b) common carotid arteries
    c) arteries   d) veins   _____

80. Blood returns to the heart from the head, face, and neck via the:
    a) common carotid   b) occipital artery
       arteries
    c) jugular veins   d) auricular artery   _____

81. The system that controls the functional activities of the glands is the:
    a) endocrine system   b) skeletal system
    c) nervous system   d) circulatory system   _____

82. Glands that lead from the gland to a particular part of the body are called:
    a) ductless glands   b) canal glands
    c) duct glands   d) channel glands   _____

83. Duct glands are also known as:
    a) endocrine glands   b) channel glands
    c) canal glands   d) exocrine glands   _____

84. Glands that release hormones directly into the
bloodstream are called:
    a) exocrine glands   b) canal glands
    c) endocrine glands   d) channel glands   _____

85. The function of the excretory system is to:
    a) circulate the blood   b) eliminate waste matter
                                 and toxins
    c) carry blood to the rest d) carry oxygen to the cells _____
       of the body

86. The gas that is expelled during exhalation from the
lungs is:
    a) carbon monoxide   b) carbon oxide
    c) carbon peroxide   d) carbon dioxide   _____

87. The greatest exchange of gases is accomplished with:
    a) shallow breathing   b) mouth breathing
    c) abdominal breathing   d) coastal breathing   _____

88. The skin and its appendages make up the:
    a) integumentary system   b) endocrine system
    c) circulatory system   d) capillary system   _____

CHAPTER 8: CHEMISTRY

1. Chemistry is the science that deals with the composition, structure, and properties of:
   - a) planning
   - b) instruction
   - c) theories
   - d) matter
   _____

2. Organic substances contain:
   - a) sodium
   - b) mercury
   - c) carbon
   - d) hydrogen
   _____

3. An example of an inorganic substance is:
   - a) metal
   - b) synthetic fabric
   - c) gasoline
   - d) plastic
   _____

4. Anything that occupies space is called:
   - a) matter
   - b) hydrogen
   - c) water
   - d) an emulsion
   _____

5. Solids, liquids, gases, and plasmas are considered to be forms of:
   - a) a substance
   - b) matter
   - c) energy
   - d) a property
   _____

6. A substance that cannot be separated into simpler substances by chemical means is a/an:
   - a) atom
   - b) compound
   - c) element
   - d) mixture
   _____

7. The smallest part of an element that retains the characteristics of that element is a/an:
   - a) elemental molecule
   - b) atom
   - c) mixture
   - d) molecule
   _____

8. When two or more atoms are chemically joined, they form a/an:
   - a) product
   - b) compound
   - c) element
   - d) molecule
   _____

9. The four types of matter are solids, liquids, gases, and:
   - a) solutions
   - b) mixtures
   - c) plasmas
   - d) compounds
   _____

10. The type of properties that can be determined without chemical reaction and change in the identity of the substance are:
    - a) chemical properties
    - b) elemental properties
    - c) physical properties
    - d) compound properties
    _____

11. Oxidation creates a change in the identity of burning wood through:
    a) physical change   b) chemical change
    c) elemental change   d) compound change   _____

12. An example of physical change is ice melting to water and:
    a) temporary haircolor   b) permanent waving
    c) permanent haircolor   d) hair straightening   _____

13. An example of a chemical change is iron to rust and:
    a) shampooing   b) rinsing
    c) permanent haircolor   d) temporary haircolor   _____

14. Elements and compounds are examples of:
    a) chemical substances   b) pure substances
    c) molecular substances   d) compromised substances   _____

15. An example of an elemental molecule is:
    a) wax paper   b) aluminum foil
    c) water   d) a pure substance   _____

16. An example of a chemical compound is:
    a) water   b) wax paper
    c) aluminum foil   d) a pure substance   _____

17. When two or more elements combine chemically, they form a/an:
    a) chemical compound   b) solution
    c) physical mixture   d) alkali   _____

18. The four classifications of compounds are acids, bases, salts, and:
    a) mixtures   b) oxides
    c) substances   d) alkalis   _____

19. When two elements combine physically, they form a:
    a) physical compound   b) solution
    c) physical mixture   d) base   _____

20. Two examples of a physical mixture are pure air and:
    a) salt   b) concrete
    c) acid   d) alkali   _____

21. The liquid that is considered to be a universal solvent is:
    a) alcohol   b) peroxide
    c) bleach   d) water   _____

22. Water is composed of:
    a) two volumes of hy-   b) two volumes of hydrogen
       drogen and one   and two volumes of oxygen
       volume of oxygen
    c) one volume of hy-   d) one volume of hydrogen and
       drogen and two   one volume of oxygen
       volumes of oxygen   _____

23. The best type of water to use in the barbershop is:
    a) distilled water   b) mineral water
    c) soft water   d) hard water   _____

24. Hard water can be softened by:
    a) freezing   b) distillation
    c) shaking   d) decomposition   _____

25. Liquid and other soaps lather easily in the presence of:
    a) soft water   b) hard water
    c) mineral water   d) an emulsion   _____

26. The pH of a liquid refers to its degree of potential:
    a) hydroxide   b) heat
    c) hydrogen   d) hardness   _____

27. The pH of a solution measures its degree of:
    a) softness or hardness   b) acidity or alkalinity
    c) heat or cold level   d) neutrality   _____

28. An ion is an atom or molecule that carries a/an:
    a) neutral charge   b) chemical charge
    c) gene   d) electrical charge   _____

29. The hydrogen ion in water is:
    a) neutral   b) alkaline
    c) acidic   d) neither a, b, or c   _____

30. The hydroxide ion in water is:
    a) neutral   b) alkaline
    c) acidic   d) neither a, b, or c   _____

31. The pH range of hair and skin is:
    a) 3.5 to 4.5   b) 4.5 to 6.5
    c) 4.5 to 5.5   d) 5.5 to 6.5   _____

32. Acidic solutions will neutralize the effects of:
    a) alkaline solutions   b) salt solutions
    c) heat or cold   d) stress on the hair   _____
       conditions

33. The chemical reaction that combines an element or compound with oxygen to produce an oxide is known as:
    a) neutralization   b) reduction
    c) oxidation   d) distillation   _____

34. The process of removing oxygen from a substance is known as:
    a) neutralization   b) reduction
    c) oxidation   d) distillation   _____

35. Hydrogen peroxide is an example of a/an:
    a) distiller   b) salt
    c) oxidizer   d) alkaline   _____

36. In a redox reaction:
    a) the oxidizer is   b) the reducing agent is
       reduced   oxidized
    c) a and b   d) neither a nor b   _____

37. A mixture of two or more substances that is made by dissolving a solid, liquid, or gaseous substance in another substance is known as a/an:
    a) solution   b) ointment
    c) suspension   d) powder   _____

38. A substance that is dissolved into a solvent is known as the:
    a) solution   b) suspension
    c) prime solvent   d) solute   _____

39. The substance that dissolves the solute is known as the:
    a) solution   b) suspension
    c) solvent   d) solute   _____

40. An example of a suspension is:
    a) a quat solution   b) hair oil tonic
    c) witch hazel   d) shampoo   _____

41. An example of an emulsion is:
    a) a quat solution   b) hair oil tonic
    c) witch hazel   d) shampoo   _____

42. Substances that act as a bridge to allow oil and water to mix or emulsify are called:
    a) bleaches   b) surfactants
    c) quats   d) solutions   _____

43. Cosmetic preparations that will cause the contraction of skin tissues are:
    a) fresheners
    b) astringents
    c) facial toners
    d) a, b, and c
    _____

44. The basic purpose of a cold cream is to:
    a) eradicate wrinkles
    b) cleanse the skin
    c) strengthen facial muscles
    d) reduce fat cells
    _____

45. Moisturizing cream causes the skin to:
    a) harden
    b) roughen
    c) soften
    d) wrinkle
    _____

46. Preparations that temporarily remove superfluous hair by dissolving it at the skin line are:
    a) depilatories
    b) epilators
    c) razors
    d) waxes
    _____

47. Preparations that remove hair by pulling it out of the follicle are a type of:
    a) depilatory
    b) epilator
    c) tweezers
    d) exfoliator
    _____

48. Scalp lotions and ointments usually contain:
    a) surfactants
    b) witch hazel
    c) alcohol
    d) medicinal agents
    _____

49. The primary ingredient in styptic powder or liquid is:
    a) talc
    b) alum
    c) alcohol
    d) witch hazel
    _____

50. Shaving soaps used in the barbershop usually contain animal or vegetable oils, water, and:
    a) zinc oxide
    b) alkaline substances
    c) acids
    d) astringents
    _____

51. Witch hazel is a solution that acts as a/an:
    a) astringent
    b) emulsion
    c) suspension
    d) acid
    _____

52. Suntan lotions are measured according to their:
    a) SPF
    b) PABA
    c) sun's rays
    d) ultraviolet rays
    _____

CHAPTER 9: ELECTRICITY AND LIGHT THERAPY

1. A form of energy that produces magnetic, chemical, or thermal effects while in motion is called:
   a) an open circuit
   b) a short circuit
   c) a broken circuit
   d) electricity
   _____

2. The flow of electricity along a conductor is known as a/an:
   a) electrical current
   b) insulator
   c) nonconductor
   d) converter
   _____

3. A substance that readily transmits an electric current is known as a/an:
   a) conductor
   b) nonconductor
   c) insulator
   d) converter
   _____

4. A substance that resists the passage of an electric current is known as a/an:
   a) converter
   b) conductor
   c) insulator
   d) rectifier
   _____

5. Rubber or silk may serve as a/an:
   a) conductor
   b) insulator
   c) electrode
   d) converter
   _____

6. A metal, such as copper wire, serves as a/an:
   a) nonconductor
   b) conductor
   c) insulator
   d) converter
   _____

7. An adjustable resistor that is used for controlling the current in a circuit is called a/an:
   a) watt
   b) ohm
   c) rheostat
   d) converter
   _____

8. A constant electrical current flowing in only one direction is called a/an:
   a) alternating current
   b) galvanic current
   c) faradic current
   d) direct current
   _____

9. An electrical current flowing first in one direction and then in the opposite direction is called a/an:
   a) direct current
   b) tesla current
   c) alternating current
   d) galvanic current
   _____

10. An apparatus that changes direct current to alternating current is called a/an:
    a) watt
    b) rectifier
    c) rheostat
    d) converter
    _____

11. An apparatus that changes alternating current to direct current is called a/an:
   a) watt   b) rectifier
   c) rheostat   d) converter   _____

12. Electric clippers and hair dryers are examples of barbering tools that use:
   a) alternating current   b) converted current
   c) direct current   d) rectified current   _____

13. Battery-operated tools such as flashlights and cordless electric clippers use:
   a) alternating current   b) converted current
   c) direct current   d) no current   _____

14. The unit that measures the pressure of the flow of electrons through a conductor is a/an:
   a) ohm   b) volt
   c) watt   d) ampere   _____

15. An ampere is a unit of electrical:
   a) pressure   b) resistance
   c) tension   d) strength   _____

13. An ohm is a unit of electrical:
   a) strength   b) pressure
   c) resistance   d) tension   _____

17. The current for facial and scalp treatments is measured in:
   a) milliamperes   b) ohms
   c) volts   d) amperes   _____

18. The amount of electrical energy being used in one second is measured in:
   a) volts   b) watts
   c) amps   d) ohms   _____

19. A safety device that prevents excessive current from passing through a circuit is a/an:
   a) circuit breaker   b) rheostat
   c) rectifier   d) fuse   _____

20. A switch that automatically shuts off an electric circuit at the first indication of an overload is a/an:
   a) circuit breaker   b) rheostat
   c) rectifier   d) fuse   _____

21. The acronym for a device that senses imbalances within an electric circuit is called a/an:
    a) OHM
    b) ECLSD
    c) PABA
    d) GFCI _____

22. All electrical appliances used in the barbershop should be:
    a) Barber Board certified
    b) FDA certified
    c) UL certified
    d) OSHA certified _____

23. The different types of currents used in facial and scalp treatments are called:
    a) units
    b) AC
    c) modalities
    d) DC _____

24. An applicator that directs electric current from the machine to the client's skin is a/an:
    a) conductor
    b) modality
    c) electrode
    d) massager _____

25. The negative or positive pole of an electric current is indicated by its:
    a) position
    b) polarity
    c) direction
    d) type of current _____

26. The positive pole is called the:
    a) anode
    b) cathode
    c) electrode
    d) direct node _____

27. The negative pole is called the:
    a) anode
    b) cathode
    c) electrode
    d) direct node _____

28. The electrical modalities available for use in barbering are galvanic current and:
    a) sinusoidal current
    b) tesla high-frequency current
    c) faradic current
    d) a, b, and c _____

29. The high-frequency current commonly used in the barbershop is the:
    a) d'Arsonval current
    b) Oudin current
    c) tesla current
    d) sinusoidal current _____

30. The tesla current is commonly called the:
    a) ultraviolet ray
    b) violet ray
    c) low-frequency current
    d) infrared ray _____

31. For a stimulating effect, the high-frequency
    electrode is:
    a) slightly lifted from   b) in close contact with
       the skin   the skin
    c) held by the client   d) turned very low   _____

32. Treatment by means of light rays is called light:
    a) therapy   b) density
    c) treatment   d) tinea   _____

33. Visible light makes up ____ % of natural sunlight.
    a) 25   b) 35
    c) 65   d) 85   _____

34. Invisible light rays make up about ____ % of natural
    sunlight.
    a) 25   b) 35
    c) 65   d) 85   _____

35. The light that produces germicidal and chemical
    benefits is the:
    a) white light   b) blue light
    c) red light   d) radiant light   _____

36. The light that produces heat and is the most penetrating
    is the:
    a) white light   b) blue light
    c) red light   d) radiant light   _____

37. Ultraviolet rays produce:
    a) heat   b) germicidal reactions
    c) chemical reactions   d) b and c   _____

38. Ultraviolet rays are also known as:
    a) actinic rays   b) cold rays
    c) tanning rays   d) a, b, and c   _____

39. Ultraviolet rays are applied:
    a) 12 to 16 inches   b) 18 to 20 inches
       from the skin   from the skin
    c) 20 to 24 inches   d) 30 to 36 inches
       from the skin   from the skin   _____

40. On average, infrared rays are applied:
    a) 12 inches from   b) 18 inches from
       the skin   the skin
    c) 20 inches from   d) 30 inches from
       the skin   the skin   _____

1. The skin covering the body is:
   a) inelastic
   b) inflexible
   c) elastic and flexible
   d) very tight _____

2. Healthy skin should be free of blemishes and:
   a) perfectly dry
   b) slightly alkaline
   c) slightly moist
   d) bluish in color _____

3. The skin is thinnest on the:
   a) eyebrows
   b) eyelids
   c) forehead
   d) back of the hand _____

4. The skin is thickest on the:
   a) palms
   b) cheeks
   c) forehead
   d) chin _____

5. The appendages of the skin are hair, nails, and:
   a) oil glands
   b) sweat glands
   c) neither a nor b
   d) a and b _____

6. The two main divisions of the skin are the epidermis and the:
   a) medulla
   b) dermis
   c) cuticle
   d) scarf skin _____

7. The outer protective layer of the skin is called the scarf skin or the:
   a) dermis
   b) adipose tissue
   c) epidermis
   d) subcutaneous tissue _____

8. Another name for the epidermis is:
   a) corium
   b) true skin
   c) cuticle
   d) derma _____

9. No blood vessels are found in the:
   a) dermis
   b) cutis
   c) subcutis
   d) epidermis _____

10. Blood vessels are found in the:
    a) epidermis
    b) dermis
    c) cuticle layer
    d) scarf skin _____

11. The color of the skin is due to the amount of blood it contains and:
    a) keratin
    b) moisture
    c) fat
    d) melanin _____

12. The layer of the epidermis that is continually being shed
    and replaced is the:
    a) stratum lucidum   b) stratum corneum
    c) stratum granulosum   d) stratum mucosum   _____

13. The stratum corneum is also known as:
    a) clear layer   b) horny layer
    c) granular layer   d) basal layer   _____

14. The epidermis contains:
    a) blood vessels   b) small nerve endings
    c) adipose tissue   d) subcutaneous tissue   _____

15. Keratin in the epidermis is found in the:
    a) stratum mucosum   b) stratum corneum
    c) stratum lucidum   d) stratum granulosum   _____

16. The stratum lucidum is also known as the:
    a) horny layer   b) grainy layer
    c) clear layer   d) reproductive layer   _____

17. The stratum granulosum is also known as the:
    a) granular layer   b) horn layer
    c) clear layer   d) reproductive layer   _____

18. The stratum germinativum is the innermost
    layer of the:
    a) dermis   b) epidermis
    c) subcutaneous   d) corium   _____

19. The growth of the epidermis starts in the:
    a) stratum lucidum   b) stratum germinativum
    c) stratum corneum   d) stratum granulosum   _____

20. The dermis is also known as the corium, cutis,
    derma, and:
    a) cuticle   b) false skin
    c) true skin   d) fatty tissue   _____

21. The reticular and papillary layers are found in the:
    a) epidermis   b) dermis
    c) cuticle   d) adipose tissue   _____

22. The papillary layer of the dermis contains looped
    capillaries and:
    a) adipose tissue   b) soft tissue
    c) subcutaneous tissue   d) nerve endings   _____

23. The reticular layer is the inner portion of the:
    a) epidermis   b) dermis
    c) cuticle   d) subcutis   _____

24. Arrector pili muscles are found in the:
    a) papillary layer   b) stratum germinativum
    c) stratum corneum   d) reticular layer   _____

25. Subcutaneous tissue consists mainly of:
    a) muscle tissue   b) fatty tissue
    c) keratin   d) pigment   _____

26. Subcutaneous tissue is also known as:
    a) muscle tissue   b) soft tissue
    c) adipose tissue   d) hard tissue   _____

27. The skin is nourished through the:
    a) blood supply   b) blood and lymph supply
    c) lymph supply   d) platelet supply   _____

28. Motor nerve fibers are distributed to the:
    a) arrector pili muscles   b) fatty tissue
    c) adipose tissue   d) fat muscles   _____

29. Sensory nerve fibers react to:
    a) hair follicles   b) freckles
    c) skin pigment   d) touch   _____

30. Secretory nerve fibers are distributed to the:
    a) sweat glands   b) oil glands
    c) neither a nor b   d) a and b   _____

31. Collagen and elastin are:
    a) sensory fibers   b) secretory fibers
    c) protein fibers   d) motor fibers   _____

32. Melanin, a skin pigment, is found in the stratum
    germinativum and:
    a) stratum corneum   b) adipose tissue
    c) papillary layer   d) reticular layer   _____

33. Melanin protects the skin from the harmful action
    of excessive:
    a) bacteria   b) pressure
    c) ultraviolet rays   d) electrical current   _____

34. The sebaceous glands are duct glands that secrete:
    a) melanin   b) saliva
    c) sebum   d) perspiration   _____

35. The function of sebum is to keep the skin:
    a) clean   b) lubricated
    c) dry   d) hard   _____

36. The duct of an oil gland empties into the:
    a) blood vessel   b) hair follicle
    c) sweat pore   d) hair papilla   _____

37. No oil glands are found on the:
    a) palms   b) face
    c) forehead   d) scalp   _____

38. The sweat glands are duct glands that excrete:
    a) sebum   b) perspiration
    c) melanin   d) oxygen   _____

39. The sweat glands help to regulate body temperature
    and eliminate _____ from the body:
    a) oxygen   b) waste products
    c) sebum   d) a and c   _____

40. The small openings of the sweat glands on the skin are
    called:
    a) follicles   b) capillaries
    c) pores   d) papillae   _____

41. The excretion of perspiration from the skin is under the
    control of the:
    a) muscular system   b) nervous system
    c) respiratory system   d) circulatory system   _____

42. Certain chemical preparations that may be absorbed into
    the skin include:
    a) antiseptic creams   b) hormone creams
    c) ointments   d) a, b, and c   _____

43. The principal functions of the skin are protection,
    sensation, heat regulation, and:
    a) excretion   b) absorption.
    c) secretion   d) a, b, and c   _____

44. Signs or indications of disease are known as:
    a) indicators   b) symptoms
    c) blemishes   d) contraindications   _____

45. Clients with an unrecognizable skin or scalp condition
    should be:
    a) referred to a   b) referred to a
       physician   pharmacist
    c) given a treatment   d) given only a haircut   _____

46. A structural change in the tissues caused by injury or disease is known as a/an:
    a) tumor   b) lesion
    c) cyst   d) fissure   _____

47. Itching is an example of a/an:
    a) subjective symptom   b) objective symptom
    c) voluntary symptom   d) imaginary symptom   _____

48. An objective symptom might look like a/an:
    a) pimple   b) boil
    c) pustule   d) a, b, or c   _____

49. Flat, nonpalpable changes in skin color, such as a macule, are characteristic of a:
    a) primary lesion   b) secondary lesion
    c) tertiary lesion   d) neither a, b, nor c   _____

50. Elevations formed by fluid in a cavity, such as a pustule, are characteristic of a:
    a) primary lesion   b) secondary lesion
    c) tertiary lesion   d) a, b, or c   _____

51. Elevated, palpable solid masses, such as a papule, are characteristic of a:
    a) primary lesion   b) secondary lesion
    c) tertiary lesion   d) neither a, b, nor c   _____

52. Examples of primary lesions include the following *except:*
    a) bulla, cyst, macule   b) vesicle, wheal
    c) papule, pustule,   d) scar, fissure, keloid   _____
       tubercle

53. An inflamed pimple containing pus is called a/an:
    a) vesicle   b) pustule
    c) macule   d) tubercle   _____

54. Poison ivy and poison oak produce:
    a) bullas   b) papules
    c) vesicles   d) tubercles   _____

55. The word that best describes a vesicle is:
    a) scar   b) abrasion
    c) blister   d) scab   _____

56. Lesions that appear as collected material on the skin or loss of skin surface are:
    a) primary lesions   b) secondary lesions
    c) tertiary lesions   d) a, b, or c   _____

57. Examples of secondary lesions include the following
   except:
   a) bulla, cyst, macule   b) scale, scab
   c) excoriation, crust   d) scar, fissure, keloid   _____

58. A thick scar resulting from excessive growth of fibrous
   tissue is called a/an:
   a) scab   b) excoriation
   c) keloid   d) crust   _____

59. The skin lesion found in chapped lips and hands is a:
   a) fissure   b) papule
   c) stain   d) tumor   _____

60. An abnormal growth of skin tissue that is usually benign
   or harmless is called a/an:
   a) tumor   b) cyst
   c) hypertrophy   d) excoriation   _____

61. The common term for keratoma is:
   a) callus   b) wart
   c) tumor   d) birthmark   _____

62. Medical attention is needed if a mole:
   a) grows in size   b) becomes sore or
      or darkens   scaly
   c) a and b   d) neither a nor b   _____

63. A skin wart is known as a:
   a) keloid   b) keratoma
   c) verruca   d) nevus   _____

64. Which of the following is not related to skin
   pigmentation?
   a) lentigines   b) hypertrophy
   c) tan   d) nevus   _____

65. Liver spots on the skin are known as:
   a) nevi   b) leucoderma
   c) chloasma   d) albinism   _____

66. A birthmark on the skin is known as:
   a) albinism   b) a nevus
   c) leucoderma   d) chloasma   _____

67. Abnormal white patches present on the skin are called:
   a) chloasma   b) albinism
   c) leukoderma   d) nevi   _____

68. The common term for lentigines is:
    a) birthmarks   b) freckles
    c) white patches   d) superfluous hair   _____

69. The general term for an inflammatory condition of
    the skin is:
    a) trichology   b) dermatology
    c) histology   d) dermatitis   _____

70. An inflammatory skin disease that may be acute or
    chronic with dry or moist lesions is:
    a) eczema   b) seborrhea
    c) psoriasis   d) herpes simplex _____

71. A chronic, inflammatory skin disease with dry red
    patches and coarse silvery scales is:
    a) eczema   b) herpes simplex
    c) psoriasis   d) dermatitis venenata _____

72. An eruptive skin infection resulting from contact with
    chemicals or tints is:
    a) eczema   b) seborrhea
    c) psoriasis   d) dermatitis venenata _____

73. A recurring viral infection that produces fever blisters or
    cold sores is:
    a) eczema   b) herpes simplex
    c) psoriasis   d) dermatitis venenata _____

74. Comedone is the technical name for a:
    a) whitehead   b) pimple
    c) blackhead   d) dry skin   _____

75. Milia is the technical name for:
    a) whiteheads   b) blackheads
    c) pimples   d) dry skin   _____

76. Acne is a disorder of the:
    a) sweat glands   b) oil glands
    c) intestinal glands d) stomach glands _____

77. A sebaceous cyst or fatty tumor that is filled with
    sebum is called a/an:
    a) steatoma   b) ulcer
    c) tumor   d) pustule   _____

78. Chronic, inflammatory congestion of the cheeks and
    nose is called:
    a) seborrhea   b) miliaria rubra
    c) sunburn   d) rosacea   _____

79. Overactivity and excessive secretion of the sebaceous
   glands may develop into:
     a) seborrhea   b) dermatitis venenata
     c) sunburn   d) rosacea   _____

80. One of the symptoms of asteatosis is:
     a) oily skin   b) clammy skin
     c) dry skin   d) warm skin   _____

81. Bromhidrosis means:
     a) lack of perspiration   b) foul-smelling perspiration
     c) excessive perspiration d) discolored perspiration _____

82. Excessive perspiration is typical of:
     a) anhidrosis   b) osmidrosis
     c) hyperhidrosis   d) bromhidrosis   _____

83. Anhidrosis means:
     a) lack of perspiration   b) excessive perspiration
     c) foul-smelling   d) prickly heat
        perspiration   _____

84. Prickly heat is the common term for:
     a) malaria fever   b) miliaria rubra
     c) ivy dermatitis   d) anhidrosis   _____

85. The most common and least severe type of skin
   cancer is:
     a) squamous cell   b) malignant melanoma
        carcinoma
     c) basal cell carcinoma   d) melanoma   _____

86. A form of skin cancer that is characterized by scaly red
   papules or nodules is:
     a) squamous cell   b) malignant melanoma
        carcinoma
     c) basal cell carcinoma   d) melanoma   _____

87. The most serious form of skin cancer, characterized by
   dark patches on the skin, is:
     a) squamous cell   b) malignant melanoma
        carcinoma
     c) basal cell carcinoma   d) melanoma   _____

88. The major factor involved in maintaining the skin's
   overall health and appearance is:
     a) heredity   b) climate
     c) diet   d) age   _____

89. The vitamin that is important to skin and tissue repair is:
     a) vitamin A   b) vitamin C
     c) vitamin D   d) vitamin E   _____

90. The vitamin that supports the overall health of
    the skin is:
     a) vitamin A   b) vitamin C
     c) vitamin D   d) vitamin E   _____

CHAPTER 11: PROPERTIES AND DISORDERS OF THE HAIR AND SCALP

1. The scientific study of hair, its disorders, and care is called:
   a) dermatology   b) trichology
   c) mycology   d) physiology   _____

2. The hair is a threadlike outgrowth of the skin present on the:
   a) palms   b) soles
   c) scalp   d) lips   _____

3. The chief purpose of hair is to:
   a) keep the scalp oily   b) protect and adorn
   c) keep the scalp dry   d) keep dandruff in place   _____

4. Hair is chiefly composed of a horny substance called:
   a) hemoglobin   b) melanin
   c) keratin   d) calcium   _____

5. Hard keratin is a substance composed of:
   a) minerals   b) protein
   c) melanin   d) chemicals   _____

6. The portion of the hair found beneath the skin surface is called the:
   a) hair root   b) hair bulb
   c) hair shaft   d) hair papilla   _____

7. The portion of the hair that extends beyond the skin surface is known as the:
   a) hair root   b) hair bulb
   c) hair shaft   d) hair follicle   _____

8. The portion of the hair that *is not* enclosed within the follicle is the:
   a) hair root   b) hair bulb
   c) hair shaft   d) hair papilla   _____

9. The main structures of the hair root are the follicle, bulb, and:
   a) dermal papilla   b) sebaceous glands
   c) arrector pili muscle   d) a, b, and c   _____

10. A tubelike depression in the skin or scalp that encases the hair root is the:
    a) hair root   b) hair bulb
    c) hair shaft   d) hair follicle   _____

11. The natural flow of the hair as it emerges from the scalp and slants in a particular direction is known as the:
    a) hair bend   b) hair structure
    c) hair stream   d) hair follicle   _____

12. A club-shaped structure that forms the lower part of the hair root is the:
    a) hair papilla   b) hair bulb
    c) hair shaft   d) hair follicle   _____

13. The structure that fits over and covers the dermal papilla is the:
    a) hair root   b) hair bulb
    c) hair shaft   d) hair follicle   _____

14. A small, cone-shaped elevation at the base of the hair follicle is called the:
    a) dermal papilla   b) hair bulb
    c) hair shaft   d) hair follicle   _____

15. Nourishment reaches the hair bulb through the:
    a) dermal papilla   b) hair root
    c) hair shaft   d) hair follicle   _____

16. Sac-like structures with ducts that are attached to each hair follicle are called:
    a) sudoriferous glands   b) sebaceous glands
    c) follicle glands   d) excretion glands   _____

17. Glands that secrete sebum to the hair and scalp are called:
    a) sudoriferous glands   b) follicle glands
    c) sebaceous glands   d) excretion glands   _____

18. Some factors that influence sebum production are:
    a) diet and blood   b) stimulated endocrine
        circulation   glands
    c) emotional distur-   d) a, b, and c
        bances and drugs   _____

19. An involuntary muscle fiber attached to the underside and base of the hair follicle is the:
    a) striated muscle   b) arrector pili muscle
    c) erector pili muscle   d) epicranius muscle   _____

20. The three main layers of the hair shaft are the:
    a) cuticle, cortex,   b) follicle, root, and bulb
        and medulla
    c) root, bulb, and   d) follicle, root, and papilla
        dermal papilla   _____

21. The outermost layer of the hair shaft is the:
    a) medulla
    b) cortex
    c) hair shaft
    d) cuticle
    _____

22. To penetrate the cuticle layer in order to reach the cortex, a solution must be:
    a) as acidic as the hair
    b) more alkaline than the hair
    c) less alkaline than the hair
    d) of a neutral pH
    _____

23. Structural changes that take place in the hair during chemical services occur within the:
    a) medulla
    b) hair shaft
    c) cortex
    d) cuticle
    _____

24. About 90% of the total weight of the hair can be traced to the:
    a) cortex
    b) shaft
    c) medulla
    d) cuticle
    _____

25. That portion of the hair that provides strength, elasticity, and natural color is the:
    a) medulla
    b) hair shaft
    c) cortex
    d) cuticle
    _____

26. The innermost layer of the hair shaft is the:
    a) medulla
    b) hair shaft
    c) cortex
    d) cuticle
    _____

27. Hair cells mature in the follicle through a process known as:
    a) cauterization
    b) dissemination
    c) keratinization
    d) propagation
    _____

28. Hair is made of approximately:
    a) 61% protein
    b) 71% protein
    c) 81% protein
    d) 91% protein
    _____

29. The elements found in human hair are carbon, oxygen, hydrogen, nitrogen, and:
    a) sulfur
    b) calcium
    c) iron
    d) glycerin
    _____

30. Proteins are made of long chains of chemical units known as:
    a) cells
    b) minerals
    c) amino acids
    d) calcium
    _____

31. Peptide bonds join amino acids:
    a) side by side   b) end to end
    c) diagonally   d) horizontally   _____

32. Peptide bonds are also known as:
    a) end bonds   b) polypeptide chains
    c) H-bonds   d) S-bonds   _____

33. End bonds are:
    a) salt bonds   b) physical bonds
    c) chemical bonds   d) hydrogen bonds   _____

34. The strongest chemical bonds in the hair are the:
    a) peptide bonds   b) salt bonds
    c) H-bonds   d) S-bonds   _____

35. Chains of joined amino acids are known as:
    a) amino chains   b) end chains
    c) chemical chains   d) polypeptide chains   _____

36. Intertwined polypeptide chains create a/an:
    a) hypertrophy shape   b) helix shape
    c) ladder shape   d) heliotrope shape   _____

37. Disulfide, hydrogen, and salt bonds are types of:
    a) cross-bonds   b) physical bonds
    c) chemical bonds   d) peptide bonds   _____

38. Approximately one-third of the hair's strength is
    attributed to the:
    a) salt bonds   b) disulfide bonds
    c) hydrogen bonds   d) a, b, and c   _____

39. Once end-bonds are broken, they can:
    a) be re-formed   b) never be re-formed
       with chemicals
    c) be fused back   d) be re-formed
       together with
       conditioners   _____

40. Disulfide bonds create:
    a) chemical cross-bonds b) cystine
    c) neither a nor b   d) both a and b   _____

41. The bonds that provide the hair with the greatest
    resistance to chemicals are the:
    a) salt bonds   b) disulfide bonds
    c) cross-bonds   d) hydrogen bonds   _____

42. Disulfide bonds may be restructured with:
    a) distilled water
    b) conditioners
    c) moisturizing shampoo
    d) certain chemical solutions   _____

43. A solution that *will not* reform disulfide bonds is:
    a) an oxidizer
    b) water
    c) hydrogen peroxide
       neutralizer
    d) a permanent wave   _____

44. Hydrogen bonds help to keep the parallel chains of polypeptides together and:
    a) add body to
       the hair
    b) keep amino acids
       connected
    c) take the place of
       salt bonds
    d) account for all
       the hair's strength   _____

45. Hydrogen bonds are:
    a) chemical bonds
    b) physical bonds
    c) mineral bonds
    d) end-bonds   _____

46. Water, dilute alkali, neutral, and acid solutions will:
    a) strengthen H-bonds
    b) increase H-bonds
    c) break H-bonds
    d) re-form H-bonds   _____

47. Drying and dilute acids will:
    a) weaken hydrogen
       bonds
    b) re-form hydrogen
       bonds
    c) dilute hydrogen
       bonds
    d) break hydrogen
       bonds   _____

48. The type of melanin that provides brown and black color to hair is:
    a) eumelanin
    b) pheomelanin
    c) dark melanin
    d) light melanin   _____

49. The type of melanin that provides a range of hair color from red to light blond tones is:
    a) eumelanin
    b) pheomelanin
    c) dark melanin
    d) light melanin   _____

50 The amount of movement in the hair strand is described as the:
    a) texture
    b) growth pattern
    c) wave pattern
    d) elasticity   _____

51. Hair growth that *is not* considered to be one of the three main types is:
    a) vellus hair
    b) primary terminal hair
    c) secondary terminal
       hair
    d) tertiary terminal hair   _____

52. Hair grows an average of:
    a) $\frac{1}{4}$ inch per month   b) $\frac{1}{2}$ inch per month

    c) $\frac{3}{4}$ inch per month   d) 1 inch per month   _____

53. It is normal to lose an average of:
    a) 25 to 50 hairs per day b) 50 to 75 hairs per day
    c) 75 to 100 hairs   d) 100 to 150 hairs per day   _____
       per day

54. Hair that flows in the same direction is known as a:
    a) hair parting   b) hair stream
    c) whorl   d) cowlick   _____

55. The hair growth pattern that forms in a circular or swirl pattern is called a:
    a) hair parting   b) hair stream
    c) whorl   d) cowlick   _____

56. Hair that protrudes straight out from the scalp may be evidence of a:
    a) hair parting   b) hair stream
    c) whorl   d) cowlick   _____

57. New hair is produced during the:
    a) anagen phase   b) catagen phase
    c) telogen phase   d) resting phase   _____

58. The transition period between the growth and resting phases of a hair strand is the:
    a) anagen phase   b) catagen phase
    c) intermediate phase d) telogen phase   _____

59. The final phase of the hair cycle that lasts until the fully grown hair is shed is called the:
    a) anagen phase   b) catagen phase
    c) intermediate phase d) telogen phase   _____

60. The anagen phase generally lasts from:
    a) one to three weeks   b) three to six months
    c) three to five years   d) one to seven years   _____

61. On average, the entire growth process of hair repeats itself once every:
    a) four or five days   b) four or five weeks
    c) four or five months d) four or five years   _____

62. To determine the hair's texture, density, porosity, and elasticity, the barber performs a/an:
    a) hair critique   b) hair analysis
    c) hair test   d) strand test   _____

63. The texture of hair that has the largest diameter is:
    a) fine hair
    b) medium hair
    c) coarse hair
    d) wiry hair
    _____

64. The term used to indicate the number of individual hair strands per square inch of scalp area is:
    a) density
    b) porosity
    c) elasticity
    d) texture
    _____

65. The ability of the hair to absorb moisture determines its:
    a) level of density
    b) level of porosity
    c) level of elasticity
    d) variation in texture
    _____

66. The ability of the hair to stretch and return to its original length without breaking is its:
    a) level of density
    b) level of porosity
    c) level of elasticity
    d) level of texture
    _____

67. Alopecia is the technical term for any abnormal type of:
    a) hair loss
    b) skin inflammation
    c) oil gland disorder
    d) sweat gland disorder
    _____

68. Hair loss that occurs as a result of genetics, age, and hormonal changes is called:
    a) androgenic alopecia
    b) alopecia senilis
    c) alopecia areata
    d) alopecia syphilitica
    _____

69. Hair loss characterized by the sudden falling out of hair in round patches is called:
    a) androgenic alopecia
    b) alopecia senilis
    c) alopecia areata
    d) alopecia syphilitica
    _____

70. Two hair loss treatments known to stimulate hair growth are:
    a) minoxidil and finasteride
    b) minoxidil and finesse
    c) minoxidil and bactericide
    d) minoxidil and ultra violet rays
    _____

71. Common scalp disorders include dandruff, vegetable and animal parasitic infections, and:
    a) diplococcal infections
    b) streptococcal infections
    c) staphylococcal infections
    d) pediculosis infestations
    _____

72. The technical term for dandruff is:
    a) alopecia
    b) steatoma
    c) pityriasis
    d) dermatitis
    _____

73. Small, white scales appearing on the scalp and hair is a sign of:
    a) dermatitis   b) eczema
    c) herpes simplex   d) pityriasis   _____

74. Classic dandruff characterized by scalp irritation, flakes, and an itchy scalp is known as:
    a) pityriasis steatoides   b) pityriasis capitis simplex
    c) psoriasis   d) dermatitis   _____

75. Dandruff characterized by accumulated greasy or waxy scales mixed with sebum is:
    a) pityriasis steatoides   b) psoriasis
    c) eczema   d) pityriasis capitis simplex   _____

76. Ringworm is an example of a/an:
    a) vegetable deficiency   b) vegetable parasitic
       disease   infection
    c) noncontagious   d) systemic infection
       infection   _____

77. Ringworm of the scalp is the common name for:
    a) tinea   b) tinea favosa
    c) tinea capitis   d) tinea sycosis   _____

78. Ringworm of the bearded area, or "barber's itch," is technically known as:
    a) tinea   b) tinea favosa
    c) tinea capitis   d) tinea sycosis   _____

79. Ringworm that is characterized by dry crusts on the scalp with a musty odor is:
    a) tinea   b) tinea favosa
    c) tinea capitis   d) tinea sycosis   _____

80. Tinea is an infection at the opening of the:
    a) sweat glands   b) oil glands
    c) blood vessels   d) hair follicles   _____

81. All forms of tinea are:
    a) nontreatable   b) contagious
    c) noncontagious   d) treatable by the
                                     barber   _____

82. Pediculosis capitis is a condition caused by:
    a) the head louse   b) the itch mite
    c) scabies   d) ringworm   _____

83. Scabies is an animal parasitic disease due to:
    a) ringworm   b) the itch mite
    c) dandruff   d) eczema   _____

84. Pediculosis and scabies are:
    a) nontreatable   b) not contagious
    c) contagious   d) treatable by the barber   _____
       infestations

85. Clients with tinea, pediculosis, or a scabies condition should be:
    a) treated by the barber   b) referred to a physician
    c) allowed barbershop   d) shampooed before
       services   haircut services   _____

86. Sycosis vulgaris, furuncles, and carbuncles are the result of a/an:
    a) diplococcal infection   b) streptococcal infection
    c) staphylococcal   d) pediculosis infestation   _____
       infection

87. A chronic bacterial infection of the follicles in the beard and mustache areas is:
    a) tinea vulgaris   b) sycosis vulgaris
    c) tinea favosa   d) tinea capitis   _____

88. The common term for a furuncle is:
    a) wart   b) milia
    c) scar   d) boil   _____

89. Inflammations of the follicle caused by bacteria or irritation may be signs of:
    a) folliculitis   b) pseudofolliculitis barbae
    c) a or b   d) neither a nor b   _____

90. When the pigment is gone and air spaces develop, the hair appears to be:
    a) black   b) brown
    c) red   d) gray   _____

91. The term that *does not* mean the development of excessive body or facial hair is:
    a) hypertrichosis   b) superfluous hair
    c) trichoptilosis   d) hirsuties   _____

92. Split hair ends are known as:
    a) congenital canities   b) trichoptilosis
    c) monilethrix   d) acquired canities   _____

93. Beaded hair is technically known as:
    a) monilethrix   b) hypertrichosis
    c) trichoptilosis   d) fragilitas crinium   _____

94. Brittle hair is technically known as:
    a) trichoptilosis   b) canities
    c) hypertrichosis   d) fragilitas crinium   _____

95. Trichorrhexis nodosa is the technical term for:
    a) knotted hair   b) split hair ends
    c) beaded hair   d) brittle hair   _____

96. The coloring pigment in the hair and skin is called:
    a) toner   b) keratin
    c) melanin   d) cystine   _____

97. "Razor bumps" is a common name for:
    a) folliculitis   b) psoriasis
    c) pseudofolliculitis   d) eczema   _____
       barbae

98. Long hair found on the scalp, beard, chest, back, and
    legs is:
    a) primary terminal hair b) secondary terminal hair
    c) tertiary terminal hair d) lanugo hair   _____

99. The term that indicates the diameter of a hair strand is
    called:
    a) hair density   b) hair porosity
    c) hair elasticity   d) hair texture   _____

100. Hair loss occurring in old age is called:
    a) androgenic alopecia   b) alopecia senilis
    c) alopecia areata   d) alopecia syphilitica   _____

CHAPTER 12: TREATMENT OF THE HAIR AND SCALP

1. The main purpose of a shampoo is to:
   a) make hair easier to comb
   b) cleanse the hair and scalp
   c) treat alopecia areata
   d) soften the scalp _____

2. Shampoo products should be selected according to the:
   a) barber's preference
   b) client's preference
   c) condition of the client's hair and scalp
   d) cost _____

3. The condition of the hair and scalp is most influenced by the shampoo product's:
   a) color
   b) acidity or alkalinity
   c) thickness
   d) lathering ability _____

4. Solutions that shrink, constrict, and harden the cuticle scales usually have a/an:
   a) acidic pH level
   b) neutral pH level
   c) alkaline pH level
   d) harsh pH level _____

5. Solutions that soften, swell, or expand the cuticle scales usually have a/an:
   a) acidic pH level
   b) neutral pH level
   c) alkaline pH level
   d) harsh pH level _____

6. Shampoo products are usually manufactured in the form of:
   a) ointments
   b) emulsions
   c) gels
   d) solutions _____

7. The usual pH range of shampoos is:
   a) 3.5 to 4.5
   b) 4.5 to 6.5
   c) 4.5 to 7.5
   d) 5.5 to 8.5 _____

8. The two main ingredients in a shampoo product are:
   a) water and soap
   b) water and surfactants
   c) soaps and oils
   d) water, buffers, and binders _____

9. The portion of the shampoo molecule that attracts water and repels dirt is the:
   a) head
   b) middle
   c) belly
   d) tail _____

10. The portion of the shampoo molecule that attracts dirt and repels water is the:
    a) head
    b) middle
    c) belly
    d) tail _____

11. Base detergents of shampoos include all of the following except:
   a) anionics b) bionics
   c) cationics d) nonionics _____

12. An anionic surfactant that is used to create a milder shampoo is:
   a) sodium laureth sulfate b) sodium lauryl sulfate
   c) cocamide d) quaternary ammonium compounds _____

13. Cocamide is a widely used:
   a) anionic surfactant b) ampholyte surfactant
   c) cationic surfactant d) nonionic surfactant _____

14. Surfactants that may be included in dandruff shampoos are usually:
   a) anionic b) ampholyte
   c) cationic d) nonionic _____

15. A type of surfactant that is used in several baby shampoos is most likely a/an:
   a) anionic b) ampholyte
   c) cationic d) nonionic _____

16. The type of shampoo that is very effective in reducing dandruff is the:
   a) green soap shampoo b) therapeutic medicated shampoo
   c) liquid dry shampoo d) egg shampoo _____

17. A shampoo formulated to prevent the stripping of permanent hair color from hair is a/an:
   a) alkaline shampoo b) medicated shampoo
   c) castile soap shampoo d) acid-balanced shampoo _____

18. Shampoos that are designed for oily hair and scalp are often:
   a) balancing shampoos b) clarifying shampoos
   c) moisturizing shampoos d) medicated shampoos _____

19. Shampoo products designed to cut through product buildup are usually:
   a) balancing shampoos b) clarifying shampoos
   c) dry shampoos d) medicated shampoos _____

20. Mild cream shampoos that contain humectants are known as:
   a) balancing shampoos
   b) clarifying shampoos
   c) moisturizing shampoos
   d) medicated shampoos
   _____

21. Special chemical agents designed to deposit protein or moisture in the hair are:
   a) shampoos
   b) conditioners
   c) styling aids
   d) scalp ointments
   _____

22. The basic types of conditioners include all of the following *except:*
   a) instant
   b) treatment or repair
   c) emulsifying
   d) leave-in
   _____

23. Finishing, detangling, and cream rinses are examples of:
   a) instant conditioners
   b) moisturizing conditioners
   c) protein conditioners
   d) leave-in conditioners
   _____

24. Conditioners that draw moisture into the hair with chemical compounds are called:
   a) deep conditioners
   b) moisturizing conditioners
   c) clarifying conditioners
   d) leave-in conditioners
   _____

25. Conditioners that penetrate the cortex to replace lost keratin are:
   a) instant conditioners
   b) moisturizing conditioners
   c) protein conditioners
   d) leave-in conditioners
   _____

26. Concentrated protein in a heavy cream base moisturizer is usually a/an:
   a) deep conditioner
   b) moisturizing conditioner
   c) clarifying conditioner
   d) leave-in conditioner
   _____

27. Leave-in conditioners:
   a) should not be rinsed out
   b) may be used with thermal tools
   c) help to equalize porosity
   d) a , b, and c
   _____

28. Rinses that are formulated to control minor dandruff and scalp conditions are:
   a) water rinses
   b) bluing rinses
   c) medicated rinses
   d) tonic rinses
   _____

29. A rinse designed to counteract yellowish or dull gray tones in the hair is a:
    a) water rinse   b) bluing rinse
    c) medicated rinse   d) tonic rinse   _____

30. A cosmetic solution that can stimulate the scalp, correct a scalp condition, or be used as a grooming aid is a:
    a) conditioner   b) styling spray
    c) hair tonic   d) scalp ointment   _____

31. The usual pH range of hair conditioners is:
    a) 2.0 to 5.5   b) 3.0 to 5.5
    c) 4.0 to 7.5   d) 6.0 to 8.5   _____

32. Shampoo and haircutting capes are two types of:
    a) shields   b) protectors
    c) drapes   d) smocks   _____

33. Nylon, cotton, or synthetic haircutting capes are preferable because they:
    a) do not require   b) are less expensive
       ironing
    c) are available in   d) shed wet or dry hair
       more colors   more effectively   _____

34. The purpose of a towel or neck strip between the drape and the client's skin is to:
    a) maintain sanitation   b) conform to state
       standards   barber laws
    c) prevent drape   d) a, b, and c
       contact with
       client's skin   _____

35. An example of a wet hair service is a:
    a) chemical service   b) shampoo service
    c) hair or scalp   d) a, b, and c
       treatment   _____

36. The two methods employed by barbers to perform a shampoo service are the:
    a) upright and reclined   b) inclined and reclined
       methods   methods
    c) tub and shower   d) backward and reclined
       methods   methods   _____

37. The most commonly used shampooing method in the barbershop is the:
    a) upright method   b) inclined method
    c) shower method   d) reclined method   _____

38. The effectiveness of a shampoo service depends on the following *except:*
    a) manner of shampoo application
    b) cost of the shampoo product
    c) quality of the scalp massage
    d) manner of rinsing

    _____

39. To determine the proper selection of shampoo and conditioning products, the barber:
    a) may analyze the hair and scalp
    b) might analyze the hair and scalp
    c) must analyze the hair and scalp
    d) should analyze the hair and scalp

    _____

40. Hair and scalp characteristics that require analysis include the following *except* the:
    a) length of the hair
    b) condition of the scalp
    c) condition of the hair
    d) porosity of the hair

    _____

41. The temperature of the water used in the shampooing process should be:
    a) cool
    b) hot
    c) warm
    d) cold

    _____

42. Shampoo and scalp manipulations are performed with:
    a) the cushions of the fingertips
    b) fingernails
    c) rubber gloves
    d) disposable gloves

    _____

43. The best time to apply scalp massage manipulations in shampooing is:
    a) before the hair has been lathered
    b) after shampoo has been rinsed
    c) after the hair has been lathered
    d) after the hair has been dried

    _____

44. Cleansing the hair without soap and water can be accomplished by using a/an:
    a) liquid dry shampoo
    b) powder dry shampoo
    c) evaporating shampoo
    d) a or b

    _____

45. The essential basic requirements for healthy hair and scalp are:
    a) cost-effective products
    b) good products and stimulation
    c) cleanliness and stimulation
    d) cleanliness and sanitation

    _____

46. A thorough scalp treatment may include cleansing, massage, and:
   a) electrotherapy
   b) light therapy
   c) tonics
   d) electrotherapy, light therapy, and tonics _____

47. Massage manipulations during the shampoo are performed with:
   a) tapping movements
   b) pinching movements
   c) scraping movements
   d) rotary movements _____

48. The blood supply to the scalp is stimulated by a/an:
   a) insulator
   b) depilatory
   c) converter
   d) scalp steam _____

49. Scalp massage should be performed with:
   a) fast motion and no pressure
   b) slow motion and no pressure
   c) continuous, even motion and pressure
   d) fast motion and heavy pressure _____

50. Barbers are qualified to perform treatments for the following *except:*
   a) dry scalp
   b) oily scalp and hair
   c) dandruff
   d) parasitic or staphylococcus conditions _____

51. The hair and scalp should be shampooed regularly to keep them free from:
   a) sebum
   b) allergies
   c) color control
   d) bacteria _____

52. Shampoo may not lather readily in hard water because the water contains:
   a) fluoride
   b) oily compounds
   c) excessive minerals
   d) distillation properties _____

53. A scalp steam *is not* used to:
   a) relax and open the pores
   b) close the pores
   c) soften the scalp
   d) increase blood circulation _____

54. Prepared steam towels may be stored:
   a) in the sink bowl
   b) on the counter
   c) in a hot towel cabinet
   d) in a plastic bowl _____

55. The purpose of a general scalp treatment is to keep the scalp and hair:
    a) lubricated   b) clean and healthy
    c) flexible   d) moisturized   _____

56. Scalp preparations containing moisturizing and emollient agents are used in:
    a) dandruff scalp   b) oily scalp and hair
       treatments   treatments
    c) dry scalp and hair   d) normal hair and scalp
       treatments   treatments   _____

57. The release of hardened sebum from the follicles is one purpose of the:
    a) dandruff scalp   b) oily scalp and hair
       treatment   treatment
    c) dry scalp and hair   d) normal hair and scalp
       treatment   treatment   _____

58. To treat a fungus condition called Malassezia, the barber may perform a/an:
    a) dandruff scalp   b) oily scalp and hair
       treatment   treatment
    c) dry scalp and hair   d) scalp treatment
       treatment   for alopecia   _____

59. A corrective hair treatment treats the:
    a) hair root   b) hair bulb
    c) hair shaft   d) hair papilla   _____

60. Scalp or hair products containing alcohol should be applied:
    a) before shampooing   b) before rinsing
    c) before applying high- d) after applying high-
       frequency current   frequency current   _____

61. Color shampoos are used for the following *except:*
    a) brightening the hair   b) creating permanent
                        color change
    c) adding slight color   d) eliminating unwanted
       to the hair   color tones   _____

62. Before applying the shampoo, dandruff may be loosened by:
    a) oiling the scalp   b) massaging the scalp
    c) steaming the scalp   d) b and c   _____

63. Instant conditioners usually have a pH that is:
    a) protein   b) alkaline
    c) acidic   d) neutral   _____

64. Protein conditioners penetrate the cortex and replace lost:
    a) acid   b) keratin
    c) moisture   d) oil   _____

65. Special conditioning formulations designed for use on badly damaged hair are:
    a) instant conditioners   b) leave-in conditioners
    c) synthetic polymer   d) moisturizing conditioners _____
       conditioners

66. Scalp massage is beneficial because it stimulates the:
    a) salivary glands   b) blood circulation
    c) pituitary gland   d) thyroid gland   _____

67. Frequent shampooing with strong soap products may cause the scalp and hair to become:
    a) fragile   b) oily
    c) dry   d) thickened   _____

68. A tight scalp can be rendered more flexible by performing a/an:
    a) egg shampoo   b) scalp massage
    c) oily scalp treatment d) scalp analysis   _____

69. Some common causes of dandruff are improper diet, uncleanliness, and:
    a) poor circulation   b) scalp manipulations
    c) oil shampoo   d) cream rinses   _____

70. A scalp treatment should never be recommended when:
    a) the scalp is healthy   b) the scalp is clean
    c) abrasions are present   d) the scalp is dry   _____

71. Nonalcoholic tonics usually contain an antiseptic solution and:
    a) hair grooming   b) styling gels
       ingredients
    c) witch hazel   d) astringents   _____

72. Alcoholic tonics containing an antiseptic and alcohol act as a/an:
    a) stimulant   b) mild astringent
    c) strong astringent   d) inhibitor   _____

73. Cream tonics are emulsions containing lanolin and:
   a) minerals
   b) astringents
   c) mineral oils
   d) alcohol
   _____

74. An oil mixture tonic is generally used as a/an:
   a) grooming agent
   b) astringent
   c) toner
   d) antiseptic
   _____

75. The value used to indicate the acidity or alkalinity of water-based solutions is:
   a) pD
   b) hP
   c) pH
   d) wB
   _____

76. When draping for a wet hair service, towels should be placed:
   a) over the cape
   b) under the cape
   c) over and under the cape
   d) on the counter
   _____

77. Instant conditioners are usually left on the hair for:
   a) 30 seconds before rinsing
   b) 1 minute before rinsing
   c) 1–5 minutes before rinsing
   d) 10 minutes before rinsing
   _____

78. One method used to treat alopecia is to:
   a) shave the head
   b) cut the hair
   c) use protein conditioners
   d) stimulate the blood supply
   _____

79. The action that *is not* caused by an acidic solution on the hair or skin is:
   a) hardening
   b) constricting
   c) softening
   d) shrinking
   _____

80. The action that is not caused by an alkaline solution on the hair or skin is:
   a) softening
   b) hardening
   c) swelling
   d) expanding
   _____

CHAPTER 13: MEN'S FACIAL MASSAGE AND TREATMENTS

1. As of 2004, the skin care clientele in spas and salons is approximately:
   a) 5 to 10% male
   b) 15 to 20% male
   c) 10 to 15% male
   d) 20 to 25% male _____

2. Regularly received facials can produce noticeable improvement in the client's:
   a) skin tone
   b) appearance of the skin
   c) skin texture
   d) a, b, and c _____

3. Three subdermal systems associated with the performance of facial treatments are:
   a) veins, arteries, and capillaries
   b) muscles, veins, and arteries
   c) muscles, nerves, and arteries
   d) veins, tissues, and nerves _____

4. When performing a facial, the types of muscles barbers need to be aware of are the:
   a) striated muscles
   b) voluntary muscles
   c) involuntary muscles
   d) nonstriated muscles _____

5. Muscles may be stimulated by:
   a) massage or electric current
   b) nerve impulses and chemicals
   c) heat and light rays
   d) a, b, and c _____

6. The epicranius muscle covers the:
   a) eyebrows
   b) top of the skull
   c) bottom of the skull
   d) cheekbones _____

7. The epicranius consists of two parts, the frontalis and the:
   a) corrugator
   b) caninus
   c) risorius
   d) occipitalis _____

8. The orbicularis oculi is a muscle that surrounds the margin of the:
   a) mouth
   b) nose
   c) eye socket
   d) head _____

9. The aponeurosis is a/an:
   a) muscle
   b) tendon
   c) nerve
   d) artery _____

10. The quadratus labii superioris is a muscle that raises and draws back the:
   a) ear
   b) eye
   c) upper lip
   d) lower lip _____

11. The orbicularis oris forms a flat band around the:
   a) eye
   b) ear
   c) mouth
   d) forehead _____

12. The mentalis is a muscle that raises the:
   a) upper lip
   b) eyelid
   c) jaw
   d) lower lip _____

13. The buccinator is a muscle that purses the:
   a) nostrils
   b) eyelids
   c) lips
   d) eyebrows _____

14. The auricular muscles are located in the:
   a) ear areas
   b) mouth area
   c) nape area
   d) cheek areas _____

15. The muscle beneath the frontalis that draws the eyebrows down and in is the:
   a) procerus
   b) buccinator
   c) corrugator
   d) mentalis _____

16. The muscle that draws the corner of the mouth out and back is the:
   a) risorius
   b) buccinator
   c) procerus
   d) mentalis _____

17. Muscles that coordinate in opening and closing the mouth are the:
   a) masseter and procerus
   b) masseter and temporalis
   c) masseter and mentalis
   d) masseter and buccinator _____

18. The muscle that allows shoulder movement and covers the back of the neck is the:
   a) trapezius
   b) risorius
   c) temporalis
   d) platysma _____

19. The sternocleidomastoideus muscle:
   a) dilates the nostrils
   b) closes the lips
   c) closes the eyes
   d) rotates and flexes the head _____

20. The muscle that is responsible for depressing the lower jaw and lip is the:
    a) trapezius
    b) risorius
    c) temporalis
    d) platysma _____

21. Stimulation to the nerves causes muscles to:
    a) expand
    b) contract
    c) expand and contract
    d) retract _____

22. Heat and moist heat on the skin causes:
    a) relaxation
    b) tightening
    c) expansion
    d) retraction _____

23. Muscles react to cold by:
    a) relaxing
    b) neutralizing
    c) contracting
    d) loosening _____

24. Nerve stimulation may be accomplished by:
    a) massage, heat, and light rays
    b) electrical current and chemicals
    c) neither a nor b
    d) a and b _____

25. Connected to parts of the brain surface, there are:
    a) 4 pairs of cranial nerves
    b) 8 pairs of cranial nerves
    c) 12 pairs of cranial nerves
    d) 16 pairs of cranial nerves _____

26. The optic nerve controls the sense of:
    a) smell
    b) sight
    c) taste
    d) touch _____

27. The olfactory nerve controls the sense of:
    a) sight
    b) smell
    c) hearing
    d) taste _____

28. The sense of hearing is controlled by the:
    a) olfactory nerve
    b) optic nerve
    c) auditory nerve
    d) facial nerve _____

29. The fifth cranial nerve is also known as the:
    a) trifacial nerve
    b) trigeminal nerve
    c) neither a nor b
    d) a and b _____

30. The trigeminal nerve is the largest and chief sensory nerve of the:
    a) occipital
    b) face
    c) chest
    d) shoulder _____

31. The motor nerve of the muscles that control chewing is the:
    a) fifth cranial nerve   b) sixth cranial nerve
    c) seventh cranial nerve   d) eighth cranial nerve   _____

32. The chief motor nerve of the face is the:
    a) fifth cranial nerve   b) sixth cranial nerve
    c) seventh cranial nerve   d) eighth cranial nerve   _____

33. Cervical nerves originate at the:
    a) occipital   b) spinal cord
    c) brain   d) trapezius   _____

34. The seventh cranial nerve is also known as the:
    a) facial nerve   b) trifacial nerve
    c) trigeminal nerve   d) cervical nerve   _____

35. The skin of the forehead and eyebrows is affected by the:
    a) supraorbital nerve   b) infraorbital nerve
    c) supratrochlear nerve   d) infratrochlear nerve   _____

36. The nerve that affects the skin of the temples, sides of the forehead, and upper part of the cheeks is the:
    a) supraorbital nerve   b) zygomatic nerve
    c) supratrochlear nerve   d) mental nerve   _____

37. The skin of the lower lip and chin is supplied by the:
    a) infraorbital nerve   b) supraorbital nerve
    c) mental nerve   d) optic nerve   _____

38. The skin of the cheek and upper lip and mouth are affected by the:
    a) infraorbital nerve   b) supraorbital nerve
    c) optic nerve   d) auricular nerve   _____

39. The temporal nerve affects the muscles of the forehead, temple, and:
    a) nose   b) upper lip
    c) lower lip   d) eyebrows   _____

40. The common carotid arteries are located at the sides of the:
    a) head   b) face
    c) neck   d) nose   _____

41. The main sources of blood supply to the head, face, and
    neck are the:
    a) spinal arteries   b) common carotid arteries
    c) occipital arteries   d) uncommon carotid arteries _____

42. The parietal artery supplies blood to the:
    a) forehead   b) back of head
    c) crown and side of   d) cheeks
       head   _____

43. The internal and external veins that serve the areas of
    head, neck, and chest are the:
    a) jugular veins   b) occipital veins
    c) carotid veins   d) auricular veins   _____

44. The external jugular vein returns the blood to the heart
    from the:
    a) brain   b) shoulders
    c) head, face, and neck   d) chest   _____

45. Conditions that may prohibit a facial massage include
    the following except:
    a) high blood pressure   b) severe skin lesions
    c) skin inflammation   d) normal skin   _____

46. A basic rule in facial massage is that any pressure should
    be applied in a/an:
    a) cross-grained direction b) upward direction
    c) downward direction   d) horizontal direction   _____

47. A point on the skin where pressure or stimulation will
    cause contraction of the muscle is a:
    a) motor point   b) trigger point
    c) sensory point   d) secretory point   _____

48. Effleurage is a massage movement is applied in a:
    a) deep rolling manner   b) tapping manner
    c) light pinching manner   d) slow and rhythmic manner
                                   without pressure   _____

49. Effleurage is used in massage for its:
    a) stimulating effects   b) soothing and relaxing
                                   effects
    c) heating effects   d) frictional effects   _____

50. Pétrissage is the type of massage movement involving:
    a) friction   b) percussion
    c) kneading or pinching   d) tapotement   _____

51. Pétrissage is used in massage for its:
    a) soothing effects   b) relaxing effects
    c) invigorating effects d) magnetic effects   _____

52. Friction in massage requires the use of:
    a) vibratory movements b) slapping movements
    c) deep rubbing   d) light stroking movements _____
    movements

53. Vibration is used in massage for its:
    a) magnetic effects   b) cooling effects
    c) soothing effects   d) stimulating effects   _____

54. Tapotement is the type of massage movement involving:
    a) vibration   b) pinching and kneading
    c) friction   d) tapping, hacking,
                               and slapping   _____

55. The immediate effects of massage are first noticed:
    a) in the mucous   b) inside the mouth
       membranes
    c) on the skin   d) under the eyelids   _____

56. Massage usually produces a/an:
    a) decrease in blood   b) increase in blood
       circulation   circulation
    c) decreased activity   d) lessened excretion
       of the skin   by skin glands   _____

57. The area of the skin being massaged reacts with a/an:
    a) increase in   b) decrease in blood
       functional activities   circulation
    c) lessened excretion   d) decreased activity
       of the skin   _____

58. Massage movements should always be directed toward
    the:
    a) insertion of muscles b) striation of muscles
    c) range of muscles   d) origin of muscles   _____

59. Massage helps to reduce:
    a) blood pressure   b) fat cells
    c) skin abrasions   d) nerve fibers   _____

60. Electrical appliances most commonly used in massage
    are:
    a) electric clippers   b) vibrators or massagers
    c) hand blowers   d) comedone extractors   _____

61. The presence of facial hair may require that massage manipulations be performed:
    a) against the hair grain
    b) across the hair grain
    c) with the grain of the hair
    d) diagonal to the hair grain _____

62. To stimulate, cleanse, and lightly exfoliate the skin a tool that can be used is a/an:
    a) vibrator
    b) brush machine
    c) electric massager
    d) cleansing cream _____

63. To warm the skin and induce the flow of oil and sweat, apply:
    a) lather
    b) vibrations
    c) steam
    d) cleansing cream _____

64. High-frequency, galvanic, faradic, and sinusoidal currents are used in:
    a) heat therapy
    b) moist-heat therapy
    c) light therapy
    d) electrotherapy _____

65. An appliance that is used to apply and direct current to the client's skin is a/an:
    a) vibrator
    b) brush machine
    c) electrode
    d) stimulator _____

66. The primary actions of the high-frequency current are:
    a) thermal and antiseptic
    b) therapeutic and antiseptic
    c) germicidal and antiseptic
    d) chemical and soothing _____

67. High-frequency electrodes are made of:
    a) glass
    b) wood
    c) metal
    d) glass or metal _____

68. Direct-surface high-frequency application requires that:
    a) the client holds the electrode
    b) the electrode is held above the skin
    c) the electrode is applied on the skin
    d) neither a, b, or c _____

69. Indirect high-frequency application requires that:
    a) the client holds the glass electrode
    b) the electrode is held above the skin
    c) the electrode is applied on the skin
    d) neither a, b, or c _____

70. General electrification using high-frequency current is performed with the:
    a) electrode applied on the skin
    b) client holding a glass electrode
    c) client holding a metal electrode
    d) electrode held above the skin
    _____

71. Do not place electrodes in an autoclave or a/an:
    a) ultraviolet ray cabinet sanitizer
    b) airtight storage case
    c) clean, closed cabinet
    d) disinfectant solution
    _____

72. Prior to a high-frequency electrical treatment, never use a skin or scalp lotion that contains:
    a) buffers
    b) alcohol
    c) cleansing agents
    d) lanolin
    _____

73. The type of machine used to produce chemical (disincrustation) and ionic (iontophoresis) reactions in the skin is a:
    a) high-frequency machine
    b) faradic machine
    c) galvanic machine
    d) sinusoidal machine
    _____

74. The disincrustation process is used to:
    a) facilitate deep pore cleansing
    b) emulsifies sebum and waste
    c) create a chemical reaction
    d) a, b, and c
    _____

75. Using galvanic current to apply water-soluble solutions into the skin layers is called:
    a) disincrustation
    b) iontophoresis
    c) phoresis
    d) cataphoresis
    _____

76. The process of forcing chemical solutions into unbroken skin using galvanic current is:
    a) anaphoresis
    b) iontophoresis
    c) phoresis
    d) cataphoresis
    _____

77. Using the positive pole to introduce an acid pH product into the skin is called:
    a) anaphoresis
    b) iontophoresis
    c) phoresis
    d) cataphoresis
    _____

78. Using the negative pole to force an alkaline pH product into the skin is called:
    a) anaphoresis
    b) iontophoresis
    c) phoresis
    d) cataphoresis
    _____

79. Ultraviolet rays are used to treat the following *except:*
   a) acne
   b) a sluggish metabolism
   c) seborrhea
   d) dandruff conditions _____

80. Increased metabolism and chemical changes within skin tissues can be achieved using:
   a) ultra violet rays
   b) infrared rays
   c) blue rays
   d) the shortest light rays _____

81. Facials performed in the barbershop are considered to be either:
   a) preventative or corrective
   b) corrective or medicinal
   c) preventative or medicinal
   d) corrective or therapeutic _____

82. In general, facial treatments are beneficial because they accomplish the following *except:*
   a) cleanse the skin
   b) tighten tense nerves
   c) increase circulation
   d) activate glandular activity _____

83. The four skin types include dry, normal, combination, and:
   a) sensitive
   b) allergic
   c) irritated
   d) oily _____

84. The stimulation of oil production and protection of the skin surface is the objective of a/an:
   a) sensitive skin facial
   b) oily skin facial
   c) dry skin facial
   d) acne skin facial _____

85. Maintenance and preventative care is the goal for:
   a) dry skin
   b) normal skin
   c) oily skin
   d) combination skin _____

86. The section of the face incorporates the forehead, nose, and chin area is known as the:
   a) oily zone
   b) T-zone
   c) dry zone
   d) sebaceous zone _____

87. Depressions in the skin that have developed from repetitious muscle action are called:
   a) scars
   b) bags
   c) wrinkles
   d) dimples _____

88. Analyzing the skin requires observation of the client's skin type and:
   a) skin condition
   b) skin texture
   c) the skin's visible appearance
   d) a, b, and c _____

89. Three essential preparations needed to perform a facial are:
    a) masks, toners, and packs
    b) cleansers, toners, and masks
    c) cleansers, toners, and moisturizers
    d) toners, moisturizers, and packs _____

90. The first cream to be used in a facial is:
    a) emollient cream
    b) tissue cream
    c) cleansing cream
    d) bleaching cream _____

91. If it should become necessary to remove the hands during facial manipulations, they should be:
    a) removed quickly
    b) feathered off
    c) removed abruptly
    d) dragged off _____

92. The sanitized end of a comedone extractor is used to remove:
    a) blackheads
    b) moles
    c) freckles
    d) birthmarks _____

93. Following the removal of blackheads, apply a/an:
    a) deodorant
    b) styptic
    c) astringent
    d) caustic _____

94. A hot-oil mask may be recommended for:
    a) oily skin
    b) dry skin
    c) tanned skin
    d) freckled skin _____

95. A clay pack should not be used for a/an:
    a) normal skin condition
    b) oily skin condition
    c) dry skin condition
    d) moist skin condition _____

96. When giving a vibratory facial, the number of vibrations should be regulated to avoid:
    a) overstimulation
    b) underrelaxation
    c) overrelaxation
    d) understimulation _____

97. A vibrator is not used over the:
    a) forehead
    b) eyebrows
    c) chin
    d) upper lip _____

98. Cleansing creams and other products should be removed from the face with a:
    a) sanitized spatula
    b) shaving brush
    c) clean, warm towel
    d) cleansing brush _____

99. Cleansing cream should be applied with:
    a) stroking and circular movements
    b) horizontal movements
    c) up-and-down movements
    d) vertical and horizontal movements
    _____

100. During a dry skin facial, the skin should not be exposed to an infrared lamp for more than:
    a) 3 minutes
    b) 5 minutes
    c) 8 minutes
    d) 10 minutes
    _____

CHAPTER 14: SHAVING AND FACIAL-HAIR DESIGN

1. When shaving a client, professional barbers use warm lather and a conventional:
   a) disposable safety razor
   b) straight razor
   c) safety razor
   d) electric razor _____

2. Individual variables that must be considered before performing a shave *do not* include:
   a) hair texture
   b) product sensitivity
   c) hair growth patterns
   d) hair color _____

3. All of the following may cause ingrown hairs *except*:
   a) excessively close shaving
   b) shear cutting
   c) excessive pressure
   d) improper use of tweezers, razor, or trimmers _____

4. When shaving a client, some states may require the use of:
   a) protective gloves
   b) goggles
   c) safety razors
   d) shaving gel _____

5. The correct angle of cutting the beard with a straight razor is called the:
   a) freehand stroke
   b) backhand stroke
   c) cutting stroke
   d) reverse freehand stroke _____

6. To achieve the best cutting stroke, the razor must glide over the surface at an angle:
   a) against the grain of the hair
   b) with the grain of the hair
   c) across the grain of the hair
   d) diagonal to the grain of the hair _____

7. The razor should be drawn in a forward movement with the point of the razor:
   a) behind the hand
   b) tilted up
   c) in the lead
   d) tilted down _____

8. The number of standard shaving positions and strokes is:
   a) two
   b) three
   c) four
   d) five _____

9. Some states may prohibit the use of:
   a) changeable-blade straight razors
   b) conventional straight razors
   c) disposable blades
   d) razor shapers _____

10. A gliding stroke directed toward the barber is used with the:
    a) freehand stroke
    b) backhand stroke
    c) cutting stroke
    d) reverse freehand stroke   _____

11. A gliding stroke directed away from the barber is used with the:
    a) freehand stroke
    b) backhand stroke
    c) cutting stroke
    d) reverse freehand stroke   _____

12. The reverse freehand position and stroke is directed:
    a) backward
    b) upward
    c) sideways
    d) diagonally   _____

13. The holding position of the razor for the reverse backhand stroke is the:
    a) same as the backhand
    b) like the reverse freehand
    c) opposite of the backhand
    d) different from the backhand   _____

14. The difference between the backhand and reverse backhand stroke is that the elbow is:
    a) positioned downward
    b) positioned upward
    c) positioned downward with forearm held upward
    d) positioned upward with forearm held downward   _____

15. Bending the wrist slightly downward while raising the elbow facilitates the:
    a) freehand stroke
    b) backhand stroke
    c) reverse freehand stroke
    d) reverse backhand stroke   _____

16. A professional shave consists of:
    a) preparation and shaving
    b) steaming and shaving
    c) preparation, shaving, and finishing
    d) shaving and finishing   _____

17. Two important steps in preparing a client for a shave are:
    a) lathering and steaming
    b) steaming and a facial
    c) lathering and finishing
    d) steaming and shaving   _____

18. Warm shaving lather is usually produced in a/an:
    a) lathering cup
    b) electric latherizer
    c) aerosol can
    d) mustache cup   _____

19. When completing each shaving movement, the once-over shave requires extra strokes:
    a) against the grain of the hair
    b) with the grain of the hair
    c) across the grain of the hair
    d) diagonal to the grain of the hair _____

20. Close shaving is the practice of shaving the beard:
    a) against or across the grain
    b) with the grain of the hair
    c) across the grain of the hair
    d) diagonal to the grain of the hair _____

21. The order in which the final steps in a facial shave should occur is:
    a) moisturize, dry, powder, and tone
    b) dry, tone, moisturize, and powder
    c) moisturize, tone, dry, and powder
    d) tone, dry, powder, and moisturize _____

22. To remove all traces of powder, lather, and loose hair, the barber uses a:
    a) blow dryer
    b) towel wrap
    c) neck strip
    d) haircutting cape _____

23. Shaving both sides of the neck below the ears and across the nape is called a/an:
    a) outline shave
    b) nape shave
    c) neck shave
    d) shave line _____

24. Lather is rubbed into the beard with the:
    a) knuckles and palms
    b) palms and wrists
    c) nail tips
    d) cushions of the fingertips _____

25. A client may find fault with a shave if the barber:
    a) wears a clean uniform
    b) has foul breath
    c) has no body odor
    d) is professional _____

26. Lathering the face for shaving serves to keep facial hairs:
    a) in an erect position
    b) flat against the skin
    c) softened in the follicle
    d) relaxed _____

27. Hot towels should not be used in the shaving procedure when the facial skin is:
    a) smooth and soft
    b) cleanly shaved
    c) chapped or blistered
    d) coarse and tough _____

28. The choice of a suitable mustache design depends on the following *except:*
    a) the client's facial features
    b) the client's personal taste
    c) the client's hair growth
    d) the barber's preference _____

29. Mustache and beard design should depend on the client's facial features and:
    a) hair growth pattern
    b) the latest trends
    c) style of the month
    d) the length of the hair _____

30. Cutting into the natural hairlines of beards and mustaches too deeply can:
    a) minimize daily maintenance
    b) decrease daily maintenance
    c) increase daily maintenance
    d) not affect daily maintenance _____

31. Men may choose to wear a beard or goatee to:
    a) balance facial features
    b) balance the face, head, and body
    c) satisfy personal preference
    d) a, b, or c _____

32. When creating a beard design line, begin:
    a) at the left sideburn
    b) in the upper cheek areas
    c) at the right sideburn
    d) in the center directly under the chin _____

33. Clipper-cut beard trims are most successful on clients whose beards are:
    a) even in density and texture
    b) fine and thin
    c) thin and coarse
    d) curly and sparse _____

34. While shaving with the dominant hand, the opposite hand stretches the skin:
    a) toward the razor
    b) away from the razor
    c) parallel to the razor
    d) diagonal to the razor _____

35. If a slight cut or scratch occurs during the shave service, apply:
    a) toner
    b) styptic powder
    c) talcum powder
    d) astringent _____

36. Mustaches should be trimmed and shaped before the following *except* the:
    a) shave service
    b) lathering process
    c) steaming process
    d) haircut service _____

37. Ingrown hairs are a common problem of:
    a) straight hair   b) wavy hair
    c) coarse hair   d) curly hair   ____

38. The number of shaving areas on the face is:
    a) 4   b) 6
    c) 14   d) 16   ____

39. The position and stroke that is most often used during a shave is the:
    a) freehand stroke   b) backhand stroke
    c) reverse freehand   d) reverse backhand stroke   ____
    stroke

40. The *final* trimming of a beard is usually performed with:
    a) a razor   b) shears
    c) an outliner   d) clipper   ____

CHAPTER 15: MEN'S HAIRCUTTING AND STYLING

1. The foundation of a good hairstyle is a good:
   - a) permanent
   - b) haircut
   - c) color
   - d) head shape _____

2. A hairstyle should accentuate the client's:
   - a) strong features
   - b) weaker features
   - c) soft features
   - d) receding features _____

3. Haircut designs require consideration of the head shape, facial contour, hairline, and the:
   - a) neckline
   - b) hair texture
   - c) neither a nor b
   - d) a and b _____

4. In addition to physical characteristics, barbers are guided in haircut design by the client's:
   - a) wishes
   - b) lifestyle
   - c) personality
   - d) a, b, and c _____

5. To eliminate any guesswork about the desired haircut or style, the barber performs a:
   - a) hair analysis
   - b) client consultation
   - c) strand test
   - d) style book presentation _____

6. Every haircut that a barber performs serves as the following *except:*
   - a) an advertisement of the work
   - b) a representation of the work
   - c) a shortcut to wealth
   - d) a possible client referral _____

7. Facial shapes are determined by the position and prominence of the:
   - a) forehead
   - b) nose
   - c) chin
   - d) facial bones _____

8. The number of facial shapes that barbers should be able to recognize is:
   - a) five
   - b) six
   - c) seven
   - d) eight _____

9. In addition to oval, round, inverted triangle, and square, general facial shapes include:
   - a) pear-shaped, oblong, diamond
   - b) rectangular, oblong, diamond
   - c) pyramid, pear-shaped, diamond
   - d) slender, rectangular, pyramid _____

10. The most recognized ideal facial shape is the:
    a) round facial shape   b) oval facial shape
    c) square facial shape   d) oblong facial shape   _____

11. Hair that is too short will emphasize the fullness of the:
    a) oval face shape   b) oblong face shape
    c) triangular face shape   d) round face shape   _____

12. Over-wide cheekbones and a narrow chin are features of the:
    a) inverted triangle   b) oval face shape
       face shape
    c) oblong face shape   d) diamond face shape   _____

13. To minimize angular features at the forehead, use
    a) deep full bangs   b) an off-the-face hairstyle
    c) wavy bangs that blend   d) bangs that cover the
       at the temples   forehead   _____

14. The facial shape that is narrow at the top and wide at the bottom is the:
    a) round   b) pear-shaped
    c) oblong   d) diamond   _____

15. When designing a hairstyle for the oblong facial shape, the objective is to:
    a) lengthen the shape   b) slenderize the shape
    c) widen the shape   d) shorten the shape   _____

16. Generally, a beard *will not:*
    a) make a face shape   b) minimize a receding
       appear oval   chin
    c) shorten the   d) widen the appearance
       appearance of the face   of a narrow jaw   _____

17. The features of a concave profile are:
    a) prominent forehead   b) receding forehead
       and chin   and chin
    c) prominent forehead   d) forehead and chin
       and receding chin   in alignment   _____

18. An arrangement of fuller hair over the forehead and a beard balances the appearance of the:
    a) straight profile   b) concave profile
    c) convex profile   d) angular profile   _____

19. To minimize a protruding chin, the client should wear a:
    a) beard only   b) mustache only
    c) long beard and   d) short beard and
       mustache   mustache   _____

20. To minimize the prominence of the nose, the hair should be styled:
    a) close and short all over
    b) forward at the front, sides back
    c) down over the forehead
    d) back at the front, down at the sides _____

21. To minimize the length of a long neck, the hair should be:
    a) left longer
    b) cut to the natural hairline
    c) cut shorter
    d) tapered close to the head _____

22. Short necks can look longer when the hair is:
    a) razor cut
    b) uniformly cut
    c) tapered
    d) left long at the nape _____

23. As part of the parietal ridge, the temporal section is also known as the following *except*:
    a) the crown
    b) the horseshoe
    c) the crest
    d) the hatband _____

24. Points on the head that mark head or hair changes as a result of the surface are called:
    a) pressure points
    b) motor points
    c) reference points
    d) trigger points _____

25. The widest section of the head is the:
    a) parietal ridge
    b) back
    c) crown
    d) sides _____

26. The bone that protrudes at the base of the skull is the:
    a) frontal bone
    b) neck bone
    c) parietal bone
    d) occipital bone _____

27. The highest point on the top of the head is the:
    a) parietal ridge
    b) back
    c) apex
    d) crown _____

28. Three types of straight lines used in haircutting are the:
    a) horizontal, vertical, zigzag
    b) horizontal, vertical, diagonal
    c) diagonal, horizontal, wavy
    d) curved, horizontal, vertical _____

29. Horizontal cutting lines:
    a) build weight
    b) reduce weight
    c) eliminate weight
    d) reduce bulk _____

30. Vertical cutting lines:
    a) increase weight   b) build weight
    c) remove weight and   d) leave weight   _____
        create layers

31. Diagonal lines produce a/an:
    a) horizontal direction   b) slanted direction
    c) parallel direction   d) opposite direction   _____

32. A space between two lines or surfaces that intersect at a given point is called a/an:
    a) line   b) angel
    c) angle   d) motor point   _____

33. The degree at which hair is held for cutting, relative from where it grows, is called:
    a) angle   b) elevation
    c) lift   d) the cutting line   _____

34. Elevation is also known as:
    a) degree   b) angle
    c) projection   d) position   _____

35. When a hair section is lifted above 0 degrees or natural fall:
    a) elevation occurs   b) blunt lines occur
    c) de-elevation occurs   d) beveling under occurs   _____

36. The outer perimeter of the cut that may act as a guideline is the:
    a) parting   b) design line
    c) elevation   d) angle   _____

37. Blunt cuts are achieved by cutting the hair at:
    a) 0 degrees   b) 45 degrees
    c) 90 degrees   d) 180 degrees   _____

38. Medium elevation creates layered ends within the parting of hair from:
    a) 0 to 90 degrees   b) 0 to 180 degrees
    c) 0 to 45 degrees   d) 0 to 360 degrees   _____

39. The most commonly used elevation used in men's haircutting is the:
    a) 0 degree   b) 45 degree
    c) 90 degree   d) 180 degree   _____

40. The usual thickness of a parting is:
    a) $\frac{1}{4}$ inch to $\frac{1}{2}$ inch   b) $\frac{1}{2}$ inch to $\frac{3}{4}$ inch
    c) $\frac{3}{4}$ inch to 1 inch   d) 1 to $1\frac{1}{2}$ inches   _____

41. The outer perimeter of the haircut is called the:
    a) guideline   b) design line
    c) cutting line   d) elevation line   _____

42. A cut by which subsequent sections of hair will be measured and cut is called a/an:
    a) guide or guideline   b) design line
    c) cutting line   d) elevation line   _____

43. Guides are classified as being either:
    a) stationary or in situ   b) moving or traveling
    c) stationary or   d) low or high   _____
       traveling

44. A guide that moves along a section of hair as each cut is made is called a/an:
    a) traveling guide   b) stationary guide
    c) mobile guide   d) universal guide   _____

45. A guide that is used to bring subsequent partings to it for cutting is called a/an:
    a) traveling guide   b) stationary guide
    c) mobile guide   d) universal guide   _____

46. Cutting the hair at elevations higher than 0 degrees produces:
    a) a blunt cut   b) a weight line
    c) layers   d) waves   _____

47. Types of layering include the following *except*:
    a) tapered layering   b) 0-degree layering
    c) uniform layering   d) angled layering   _____

48. A haircut that conforms to the shape of the head is usually:
    a) blunt cut   b) uniformly cut
    c) tapered   d) long layered   _____

49. A tapered haircut is longer in the crown and top areas and:
    a) shorter at the nape   b) uniform at the nape
    c) longer at the nape   d) neither a, b, or c   _____

50. The heaviest perimeter area of a 0- or 45-degree cut may be referred to as a:
    a) cutting line   b) bowl cut line
    c) weight line   d) bi-level line   _____

51. The use of barbering tools to create special effects within a haircut is called:
    a) specializing
    b) texturizing
    c) layering
    d) slithering _____

52. The amount of pressure applied to the hair while combing or holding for cutting is called:
    a) stretching
    b) controlling
    c) tension
    d) texturizing _____

53. The removal of excess bulk from the hair is called:
    a) slithering
    b) dethickening
    c) customizing
    d) thinning _____

54. Marking or finishing the outer perimeter of the haircut is called the following *except*:
    a) outlining
    b) bordering
    c) edging
    d) a tape-up _____

55. Combing the hair away from its natural fall position for cutting results in:
    a) underdirection
    b) overdirection
    c) angled-direction
    d) neither a, b, nor c _____

56. Hairstyling may require one of the following *except*:
    a) oil sheen
    b) hair tonic
    c) styling gel
    d) styptic _____

57. Cutting-above-the-fingers is a:
    a) fingers-and-shear technique
    b) shear-over-comb technique
    c) free-hand technique
    d) razor-rotation technique _____

58. An important haircutting technique used in tapering is the:
    a) fingers-and-shear technique
    b) shear-over-comb technique
    c) universal technique
    d) free-hand shear technique _____

59. Using the shear-over-comb method to cut behind the ears may require the comb to be in a:
    a) vertical position
    b) horizontal position
    c) diagonal position
    d) position atop the hair _____

60. When using the shear-over-comb technique, the comb is held parallel to the:
    a) hairline
    b) shears
    c) part line
    d) hair clip _____

61. When using the shear-over-comb technique, the hair is placed in position for cutting by:
    a) combing through it
    b) holding hair between the fingers
    c) brushing through the hair
    d) rolling the comb out   _____

62. The shear point taper is performed with the:
    a) cutting points of the shears
    b) razor
    c) clippers
    d) outliners   _____

63. Marking the outer border of the haircut along the curved areas of the hairline is called the:
    a) outlining technique
    b) trimming technique
    c) arching technique
    d) finishing technique   _____

64. The standard clipper cutting techniques are the:
    a) freehand and backhand
    b) clipper-over-comb and freehand
    c) freehand and underhand
    d) clipper-over-comb and backhand   _____

65. As a general rule, clipper cutting is followed up with:
    a) razor rotation work
    b) trimmer work
    c) shear work
    d) comb and shear work   _____

66. Cutting *against the grain* means to cut the hair in the direction:
    a) opposite from which it grows
    b) diagonal from which it grows
    c) that it grows
    d) neither a, b, or c   _____

67. If the barber is not cutting in an upward or downward direction with the clippers, he/she is probably cutting the hair:
    a) against the grain
    b) across the grain
    c) with the grain
    d) opposite the grain   _____

68. Cutting the hair in a circular motion with the grain is advisable in areas where:
    a) cowlicks are present
    b) waves are present
    c) whorls are present
    d) whirls are present   _____

69. Free-hand clipper cutting requires consistent use of the:
    a) comb or hair pick
    b) outliner
    c) trimmer
    d) edger   _____

70. The usual range of detachable clippers blades range is 0000 to size:
    a) 1
    b) 2
    c) 3
    d) $3\frac{1}{2}$ _____

71. To blend a taper from shorter to longer hair using the clipper-over-comb method:
    a) place the comb flat to the head
    b) tilt the comb toward the head
    c) tilt the comb away from the head
    d) freehand blend the hair _____

72. Fades, crew cuts, flat tops, and the Quo Vadis are examples of popular:
    a) shear cuts
    b) clipper cuts
    c) razor cuts
    d) trimmer cuts _____

73. Always check sideburn lengths by:
    a) facing the client
    b) measuring from facial bones
    c) measuring from the ear
    d) facing the client toward the mirror _____

74. The type of cutting method that can help make resistant hair textures more manageable is:
    a) clipper cutting
    b) razor cutting
    c) shear cutting
    d) hair singeing _____

75. The razor is held almost flat against the surface of the hair in:
    a) light taper-blending
    b) terminal taper-blending
    c) razor taper-blending
    d) heavy taper-blending _____

76. The razor is held up to 45 degrees from the surface of the hair strand in:
    a) light taper-blending
    b) terminal taper-blending
    c) razor taper-blending
    d) heavy taper-blending _____

77. The angle of the razor blade is increased to about 90 degrees in:
    a) light taper-blending
    b) terminal taper-blending
    c) razor taper-blending
    d) heavy taper-blending _____

78. Hair that requires more razor strokes and heavier tapering than other textures is:
    a) fine, thick hair
    b) coarse, thick hair
    c) medium, thick hair
    d) any thick hair type _____

79. The rotating motion of the comb and razor as the hair is being cut is called:
    a) cutting rotation b) slicing rotation
    c) razor rotation d) razor taper-blending _____

80. Razor cutting requires that the hair be:
    a) chemically processed b) clean and damp
    c) clean and dry d) misted _____

81. When thinning the hair, avoid the following *except:*
    a) cutting too deeply b) cutting too close to the scalp
    c) cutting top surfaces of the hair d) observation of area to be thinned _____

82. The neck shave and shaving of the outline areas are considered to be the following *except:*
    a) unnecessary b) traditional barbering services
    c) haircut finish work d) important to the finished cut _____

83. Shaving the sides of the neck and across the nape with a razor is called a/an:
    a) extra service b) outline shave
    c) neck shave d) hairline shave _____

84. The arranging the hair into an appropriate style following a haircut or shampoo is called:
    a) hair arranging b) hairstyling
    c) hair sculpting d) hair finishing _____

85. Blow-drying techniques include the following *except:*
    a) free-form b) stylized
    c) diffused d) thermal irons _____

86. One of the most popular braiding variations chosen by men are:
    a) fish-bone braid b) on-the-scalp cornrows
    c) three-strand braid d) off-the-scalp cornrows _____

87. Styling the hair into braids and locks is a form of:
    a) natural hair care b) chemical hair care
    c) trendy hair care d) thermal hair care _____

88. The process that occurs when coily hair is allowed to develop in its natural state is called:
    a) natural hair b) braiding
    c) hairlocking d) corn-rowing _____

89. Once locked, locks can be removed only by:
    a) cutting them off   b) chemical processes
    c) shampooing   d) shampooing and
                                  conditioning   _____

90. Hair locks in progressive stages that can take
    a) 1 to 3 months   b) 3 to 6 months
       to complete   to complete
    c) 6 to 9 months   d) 6 to 12 months to
       to complete   complete   _____

91. Techniques for locking the hair include the following
    except:
    a) curling iron method   b) comb revolution
                                  blending
    c) finger-rolling method   d) palm-rolling method   _____

92. Hair thinning is used primarily for:
    a) shortening hair   b) difficult hair types
       length
    c) whorl sections of hair d) reducing bulk in the hair _____

93. A style suitable for very curly hair that is even over the
    entire head is the:
    a) fade style   b) precisioncut style
    c) Quo Vadis style   d) brushcut style   _____

94. In shear-over-comb cutting, the comb is held parallel to
    the:
    a) still blade of   b) forearm of the barber
       the shears
    c) client's neckline   d) cutting blade of the shears _____

95. A special clipper designed primarily for close cutting in
    the outline areas is called a/an:
    a) razor   b) balding clipper
    c) edger, trimmer or   d) vibrator
       outliner   _____

96. In razor cutting, the type of razor that is preferable for
    beginning barbers is the:
    a) electric razor   b) wedge razor
    c) open-blade razor   d) guarded razor   _____

97. For best results in razor cutting the barber must avoid:
    a) tapering and   b) overtapering
       blending
    c) ear arching   d) blunt cutting   _____

98. The best results occur in finger waving when the hair:
    a) is straight
    b) is short
    c) has a natural or
       permanent wave
    d) artificially colored _____

99. Finger waving requires the following items *except:*
    a) comb and hair net
    b) curling iron
    c) waving or styling
       lotion
    d) hairpins or clips _____

100. The ridges in a shadow wave are:
     a) lower than a
        finger wave ridge
     b) higher than a
        finger wave ridge
     c) the same as a
        finger wave ridge
     d) neither a, b, or c _____

CHAPTER 16: MEN'S HAIRPIECES

1. During the eighteenth century, *toupee* described the front section of hair known as the:
   a) apex
   b) crown
   c) foretop
   d) queue   _____

2. Today, a small hairpiece or wig used to cover the top or crown of the head is called a:
   a) wiglet
   b) toupee
   c) full-bottom wig
   d) periwig   _____

3. The primary purpose for wearing a hairpiece is to:
   a) change hair color
   b) maintain cleanliness
   c) cover baldness
   d) look older   _____

4. Hair replacement techniques include toupees or hairpieces and the following *except:*
   a) certain drugs
   b) chemical processes
   c) surgical hair transplantation
   d) scalp reduction   _____

5. The quality of a hairpiece varies with the kind of hair used in its manufacture and its:
   a) manner of construction
   b) color
   c) fit
   d) shape   _____

6. The most desirable choice for a quality hairpiece is:
   a) synthetic hair
   b) animal hair
   c) mixed hair products
   d) human hair   _____

7. Advantages of human hair hairpieces include the following *except:*
   a) more natural look and texture
   b) more rapid fading
   c) tolerance of chemical processes
   d) durability   _____

8. Disadvantages associated with a human hair hairpiece include the following *except:*
   a) reacts to climate changes
   b) requires styling maintenance
   c) its natural look
   d) becomes damaged the same as natural hair   _____

9. A significant amount of the human hair used in hairpieces comes from:
   a) Russia and Europe   b) Europe and Asia
   c) the United States   d) Europe and Australia   _____
   and Europe

10. Hairpieces made of human hair must be:
    a) shampooed and   b) dry cleaned
    conditioned
    c) washed with   d) cleaned with acetone   _____
    warm water

11. Synthetic hair is used primarily in the production of:
    a) full wigs   b) men's hairpieces
    c) toupees   d) false mustaches   _____

12. Characteristics of synthetic fibers used in hairpieces or wigs include the following *except:*
    a) a high gloss   b) tend to mat and tangle
    c) must be dry cleaned   d) difficult to blend with   _____
    natural hair

13. Animal hair used to manufacture of wigs and hairpieces include the following *except:*
    a) cat hair   b) sheep's wool
    c) angora hair   d) yak hair   _____

14. Synthetic hairpieces are usually cleaned with:
    a) acetone   b) dry-cleaning solvent
    c) shampoo and water   d) water only   _____

15. Bases that are available for hairpieces include hard, soft, mesh, net, polyurethane, and:
    a) three-fold bases   b) combination bases
    c) stacked bases   d) wedged bases   _____

16. Standard types of hairpiece construction include the following *except:*
    a) wefted   b) soft or hard base
    c) hand-sewn,   d) laser driven   _____
    hand-tied

17. Custom hairpieces require the following *except:*
    a) color matching   b) measurements
    c) a stock size   d) a pattern   _____
    for each client

18. A hairpiece pattern analysis is also known as a:
    a) shape analysis   b) size analysis
    c) contour analysis   d) form analysis   _____

19. Cuttings from the client's natural hair are used as a:
    a) texture and   b) color and
       color guide   length guide
    c) texture and   d) color and
       size guide   thickness guide   _____

20. The sizes of men's hairpieces are commonly measured in:
    a) millimeters   b) inches
    c) centimeters   d) kilometers   _____

21. A lace-front hairpiece is recommended when the hair is
    worn:
    a) in an off-the-   b) down over the
       face style   forehead
    c) with a right side part d) with a left side part _____

22. Hairpieces may be cut and blended with shears or a/an:
    a) clipper   b) outliner
    c) razor   d) edger   _____

23. Two methods for attaching a hairpiece are:
    a) weft glue and tape   b) double-sided tape and
                               spirit gum
    c) tape and glue   d) spirit gum and weft glue _____

24. When a hairpiece is not being worn, it should be placed
    on a/an:
    a) head mold   b) hook
    c) wig block   d) flat surface   _____

25. Displays, referrals, print ads, and the personal approach
    are examples of:
    a) record keeping   b) marketing techniques
    c) business management d) business savvy   _____

26. Forms of surgical hair restoration include the following
    except:
    a) toupees   b) scalp reduction
    c) hair transplantation d) flap surgery   _____

27. A topical medication for hair loss manufactured under
    different brand names is:
    a) ether   b) minoxidil
    c) mineral oil   d) hair tonic   _____

28. Hair weaving is a form of:
    a) wig making
    b) surgical hair restoration
    c) surgical hair replacement
    d) nonsurgical hair replacement   _____

29. Before removing a lace-front hairpiece, dampen the lace with:
    a) water
    b) acetone or solvent
    c) kerosene
    d) alcohol   _____

30. Permanent waving and haircoloring services may be performed on:
    a) human hair hairpieces
    b) synthetic hairpieces
    c) yak hair hairpieces
    d) horse hair hairpieces   _____

31. Facial hairpieces are usually applied with:
    a) acetone
    b) spirit gum
    c) tape
    d) weft glue   _____

32. Used in the production of wigs, kanekalon, dynel, and venicelon are:
    a) natural hair fibers
    b) animal hair fibers
    c) modacrylic fibers
    d) human hair fibers   _____

33. A hairpiece should never be:
    a) combed
    b) folded
    c) cut
    d) styled   _____

34. Reconditioning treatments for hairpieces:
    a) take the place of cleaning
    b) should take place weekly
    c) prevent dryness or brittleness of the hair
    d) are not required   _____

35. The foundation of a hair weave must be tightened and brought close to the scalp every:
    a) week
    b) two to four weeks
    c) two weeks
    d) four to eight weeks   _____

CHAPTER 17: WOMEN'S HAIRCUTTING AND STYLING

1. Most women's styles require:
   - a) less styling than men's styles
   - b) the same styling as men's styles
   - c) more styling than men's styles
   - d) neither a, b, or c
   _____

2. The four basic haircuts are the blunt, graduated, uniform layers, and:
   - a) tapered
   - b) stacked
   - c) long layers
   - d) short layers
   _____

3. The haircut that *looks* like all the hair is the same length is the:
   - a) blunt cut
   - b) long layered cut
   - c) graduated cut
   - d) uniform layer cut

4. If the head is tilted forward while cutting the nape during a blunt cut, it will create:
   - a) high-elevation layering
   - b) graduation
   - c) uniform layering
   - d) no change within the cut
   _____

5. A graduated cut has a wedge shape that is created by cutting with tension at:
   - a) low to high elevations
   - b) low to very high elevations
   - c) medium to high elevations
   - d) low to medium elevations
   _____

6. Maintain uniform moisture in the hair while:
   - a) styling
   - b) cutting
   - c) drying
   - d) combing
   _____

7. When cutting the hair at 90 degrees, the hair is projected 90 degrees from:
   - a) the hairline
   - b) the previous section
   - c) where it grows
   - d) the widest part of the head form
   _____

8. When cutting hair from one section to the next, always use a:
   - a) guide
   - b) strand test
   - c) light comb
   - d) dark comb
   _____

9. More volume will be created within the cut if:
   - a) thick partings are used
   - b) medium-thick partings are used
   - c) thin partings are used
   - d) no partings are used
   _____

10. To achieve a long layered cut, the hair is projected and cut at:
    a) 0 degrees
    b) 45 degrees
    c) 90 degrees
    d) 180 degrees
    _____

11. When layering the hair, the hanging length to remain can be better controlled by:
    a) cutting the top section
    b) creating uniform layers
    c) cutting in the layers first
    d) cutting the perimeter design line first
    _____

12. Sections within a haircut can be blended:
    a) from short to long
    b) from long to short
    c) neither a nor b
    d) a and b
    _____

13. Wavy and curly hair have the following characteristics *except:*
    a) wave troughs
    b) straight ends
    c) wave crests
    d) elasticity
    _____

14. When cut at low elevations, wavy and curly hair tends to:
    a) bevel under
    b) bevel up
    c) graduate naturally
    d) straighten
    _____

15. Cutting just after the wave crest as it dips toward the trough may encourage the hair to:
    a) fall inward toward the head form
    b) curl more tightly
    c) flip outward away from the head form
    d) straighten
    _____

16. When cutting curly hair, after each cut with the clipper, comb or pick the hair to:
    a) detangle the hair
    b) check the cutting effect
    c) thin the hair
    d) thicken the hair
    _____

17. Razor cutting produces an angle at the ends of the hair that results in:
    a) blunt-shaped hair ends
    b) curls
    c) soft shapes with movement
    d) soft shapes with no movement
    _____

18. The most commonly used texturizing techniques is/are:
    a) point cutting
    b) slicing and carving
    c) notching and slithering
    d) a, b, and c
    _____

19. Two texturizing techniques that are performed on the hair ends are:
    a) point cutting and notching
    b) slicing and carving
    c) notching and slithering
    d) slicing and notching _____

20. The wet setting method that uses the client's head as a form or tool is a:
    a) pin curl
    b) roller set
    c) hair wrapping
    d) Velcro roller set _____

21. Wet-setting techniques include the following *except:*
    a) pin curls
    b) finger waves
    c) hair wrapping
    d) thermal-iron work _____

22. When blow-drying the hair, begin in the:
    a) nape area
    b) back area
    c) top area
    d) side areas _____

23. To blow-dry short, curly hair into its natural wave pattern use a:
    a) comb attachment
    b) diffuser attachment
    c) nozzle attachment
    d) brush attachment _____

24. Using heat to produce waving or straightening effects is known as:
    a) roller setting
    b) wet styling
    c) thermal styling
    d) dry styling _____

25. Thermal waving is achieved with:
    a) rollers
    b) marcel or curling irons
    c) perm rods
    d) pressing combs _____

26. Thermal straightening can be achieved with:
    a) curling irons
    b) electric flat irons
    c) pressing combs
    d) b and c _____

27. The projection of the hair from the scalp will determine where the curl sits in relation to its:
    a) base
    b) circle
    c) stem
    d) curl _____

28. The foundation on which the curling iron barrel or a roller is placed is called the:
    a) base
    b) stem
    c) curl
    d) circle _____

29. The part of a curl that gives the hair direction and mobility is the:
   a) base b) circle
   c) stem d) curl _____

30. The three types of bases used in thermal and roller setting are:
   a) on-base, off-base, half off-base
   b) off-base, half on-base, on-base
   c) on-base, off-base, quarter-base
   d) neither a, b, nor c _____

31. Hair pressing straightens extremely curly hair:
   a) using chemicals b) temporarily
   c) permanently d) not at all _____

32. About 50 to 60% of the curl will be removed with a:
   a) hard press b) oiled press
   c) soft press d) medium press _____

33. To prevent the hair from burning or scorching during pressing, apply a/an:
   a) pressing cream b) oil
   c) astringent d) a or b _____

34. About 100% of the curl will be removed with a:
   a) hard press b) oiled press
   c) soft press d) medium press _____

35. Apply the pressing comb twice on each side of the hair section for a/an:
   a) oiled press b) soft press
   c) hard press d) medium press _____

CHAPTER 18: CHEMICAL TEXTURE SERVICES

1. Chemical texture services create chemical changes in the hair that are:
   - a) temporary
   - b) permanent
   - c) occasional
   - d) neither a, b, or c
   _____

2. Chemical texture services include the following *except:*
   - a) reformation curls
   - b) hair relaxing
   - c) permanent waving
   - d) hair coloring
   _____

3. When new hair growth occurs, changes in the hair created by chemical services require a:
   - a) redo service to maintain
   - b) reverting service to maintain
   - c) retouch service to maintain
   - d) reaction service to maintain
   _____

4. The process used to chemically restructure straight hair into a wave pattern is:
   - a) permanent waving
   - b) haircoloring
   - c) reformation curls
   - d) hair relaxing
   _____

5. Permanent waving requires the use of the following *except:*
   - a) rods
   - b) neutralizer
   - c) a waving lotion
   - d) rearranger
   _____

6. A reformation curl is also known as the following *except:*
   - a) chemical blow-out
   - b) Jheri curl
   - c) soft-curl perm
   - d) a curl
   _____

7. A relaxing product that is used to partially straighten the hair is required for a:
   - a) permanent wave
   - b) haircolor
   - c) reformation curl
   - d) chemical hair relaxing
   _____

8. The process used to chemically restructure curly hair into a larger curl pattern is called a:
   - a) reformation curl
   - b) roller set
   - c) permanent wave
   - d) hair relaxing
   _____

9. The process used to rearrange overcurly hair into a straightened hair form is known as:
   - a) permanent wave
   - b) a curl
   - c) reformation curl
   - d) chemical hair relaxing
   _____

10. The two layers of the hair most affected by chemical texture services are the:

    a) cortex and medulla   b) cortex and cuticle

    c) medulla and cuticle   d) cortex and hair root   _____

11. The degree to which hair is resistant to chemical changes depends on the strength of the:

    a) cuticle   b) hair shaft

    c) hair root   d) medulla   _____

12. Alkaline solutions used in chemical texture services soften and swell the:

    a) medulla   b) cuticle

    c) cortex   d) hair follicle   _____

13. Through softening and swelling, alkaline solutions facilitate penetration into the:

    a) medulla   b) hair follicle

    c) hair root   d) cortex   _____

14. The hair's strength, flexibility, elasticity, and shape are found in the:

    a) medulla   b) cuticle

    c) cortex   d) hair follicle   _____

15. Chemical bonds in the hair are broken or rearranged by:

    a) physical changes   b) roller setting

    c) chemical services   d) blow-drying   _____

        and processes

16. Cysteine is an amino acid created by:

    a) the reduction   b) the reduction of

        of cystine   hydrogen bonds

    c) physical processes   d) the reduction of

                                  salt bonds   _____

17. Cysteine is changed back to the cystine state during the process of oxidation and:

    a) processing   b) neutralization

    c) reduction   d) softening and swelling   _____

18. The two principal actions on the hair during a chemical texture service are:

    a) softening and   b) swelling and constricting

        hardening

    c) expansion and   d) physical and chemical   _____

        contraction

19. The physical actions involved in permanent waving include the following *except:*
    a) shampooing
    b) neutralizing
    c) rinsing
    d) rodding
    _____

20. Chemical actions take place within a permanent wave process during:
    a) processing
    b) neutralizing
    c) rearranging
    d) a and b
    _____

21. In permanent waving, the waving lotion is also known as a/an:
    a) neutralizer
    b) developer
    c) reducing agent
    d) oxidizer
    _____

22. Neutralizers rebond rearranged disulfide bonds through a process known as:
    a) oxidation
    b) processing
    c) reducing
    d) pH balancing
    _____

23. The reformation curl service requires the physical actions of the following *except:*
    a) shampooing
    b) rearranging
    c) combing
    d) rodding
    _____

24. Chemical actions involved in a reformation curl are facilitated by the following, *except:*
    a) rearranger
    b) neutralizer
    c) booster
    d) leave-in conditioner
    _____

25. The primary difference between permanent waving lotion and a rearranger is a matter of:
    a) color
    b) cost
    c) consistency
    d) compatibility
    _____

26. Rearrangers are:
    a) thinner than waving lotions
    b) thicker than waving lotions
    c) more translucent than waving lotions
    d) the same consistency as waving lotions
    _____

27. The neutralizing process of reformation curls is:
    a) different from permanent waving
    b) the same as permanent waving
    c) a and b
    d) neither a nor b
    _____

28. The hair-relaxing process requires the physical actions of the following *except:*
   a) combing and smoothing
   b) shampooing and rinsing
   c) rodding
   d) conditioning _____

29. The primary chemical action that occurs in hair relaxing is the result of the:
   a) relaxing product
   b) shampoo
   c) combing
   d) conditioner _____

30. Hydroxide relaxing products are neutralized through the process of:
   a) oxidizing
   b) neutralization
   c) shampooing and rinsing
   d) conditioning _____

31. Hydroxide relaxers and thio relaxers are:
   a) compatible
   b) not compatible
   c) interchangeable
   d) the same _____

32. The permanent breaking of disulfide bonds with a hydroxide relaxer is called:
   a) oxidation
   b) lanthionization
   c) neutralization
   d) reduction _____

33. Ammonium thioglycolate relaxers use an oxidizing agent such as:
   a) water
   b) prewrap lotion
   c) waving lotion
   d) hydrogen peroxide _____

34. Disulfide bonds broken by a hydroxide relaxer:
   a) cannot be re-formed
   b) can be bonded
   c) are temporarily rearranged
   d) are repairable _____

35. Before proceeding with any chemical service, the barber must determine the:
   a) client's expectations
   b) hair type and its condition
   c) degree to which expectations can be met
   d) a, b, and c _____

36. Information learned during the consultation should be recorded on a/an:
   a) appointment book
   b) in a log book
   c) client record card
   d) client list _____

37. A chemical service should not be given if the scalp shows signs of:
    a) cuts
    b) abrasions
    c) lesions
    d) a, b, and c
    _____

38. A chemical service should not be given if the hair shows signs of:
    a) porosity
    b) elasticity
    c) overporosity and breakage
    d) nonporosity
    _____

39. Hair with a tight, compact cuticle layer is considered to be:
    a) resistant
    b) normal porous
    c) porous
    d) overporous
    _____

40. Hair that has a raised cuticle layer that easily absorbs solutions is considered to be:
    a) resistant
    b) normal porous
    c) porous
    d) overporous
    _____

41. Sliding the fingers along a strand of hair from the ends to the scalp is called a:
    a) strand test
    b) pull test
    c) relaxer test
    d) porosity test
    _____

42. Hair analysis for chemical texture services include the hair's porosity, texture, and:
    a) direction of hair growth
    b) density
    c) length
    d) a, b, and c
    _____

43. Hair texture describes the diameter of a strand of hair as being all of the following except:
    a) fine
    b) thick
    c) coarse
    d) medium
    _____

44. The hair's elasticity is an indication of the strength of its:
    a) medulla
    b) cuticle
    c) cross-bonds
    d) diameter
    _____

45. Hair density is analyzed to determine the thickness of subsections, the size of rods, and the:
    a) amount of product to use
    b) elasticity of the hair
    c) porosity level of the hair
    d) texture of the hair
    _____

46. The two principal actions involved in permanent waving are:
    a) rodding and wrapping
    b) physical and chemical
    c) shampooing and rinsing
    d) neither a, b, or c
    _____

47. In permanent waving, wrapping the hair around the rods is a/an:
    a) optional action
    b) unnecessary action
    c) chemical action
    d) physical action
    _____

48. The two chemical actions that take place in permanent waving are:
    a) rodding and wrapping
    b) physical and chemical
    c) processing and neutralizing
    d) shampooing and rinsing
    _____

49. The size of the waving rod determines the size of the:
    a) curl or wave
    b) end paper
    c) solution bottle
    d) comb used
    _____

50. Concave, straight, bender, and loop refer to types of:
    a) end wraps
    b) rollers
    c) perm rods
    d) hair clips
    _____

51. Absorbent papers that are used to control the ends of the hair while rodding are called:
    a) end wraps
    b) end papers
    c) neither a nor b
    d) a and b
    _____

52. Common end paper–wrapping techniques include the following *except:*
    a) bookend wrap
    b) double end wrap
    c) single flat or single end wrap
    d) double bookend wrap
    _____

53. A parting taken from the subsection that is rodded or wrapped is called:
    a) base section
    b) parting
    c) section
    d) working panel
    _____

54. The position of the perm rod or tool in relation to its base section is called:
    a) base section
    b) section
    c) base control
    d) working panel
    _____

55. The hair is projected about 45 degrees beyond 90 degrees to its base section in a/an:
    a) off-base rod placement
    b) on-base rod placement
    c) half off-base rod placement
    d) any rod placement _____

56. Wrapping the hair at an angle of 90 degrees to its base section results in:
    a) off-base rod placement
    b) on-base rod placement
    c) half off-base rod placement
    d) quarter-off rod placements _____

57. Rodding the hair at a 45-degree angle below 90 degrees to its base section produces:
    a) off-base rod placement
    b) on-base rod placement
    c) half-off-base rod placement
    d) any rod placement _____

58. The directional pattern in which the hair is rodded or wrapped is called the:
    a) base point
    b) base pattern
    c) base section
    d) base direction _____

59. Two basic methods used to wrap the hair around the perm rod are the:
    a) croquignole and spiral
    b) basic and croquignole
    c) spiral and underhand
    d) overhand and spiral _____

60. The standard method used to wind the hair from the ends toward the scalp is the:
    a) basic method
    b) croquignole method
    c) overhand method
    d) underhand method _____

61. Two wrapping methods used in permanent waving are the:
    a) setting lotion and water wraps
    b) neutralizer and water wraps
    c) lotion and water wraps
    d) conditioner and water wraps _____

62. The application of waving solution to a section of hair just prior to rodding is the:
    a) water wrap
    b) neutralizer wrap
    c) lotion wrap
    d) conditioner wrap _____

116

63. Characteristics of the lotion wrap include the following *except:*
    a) presoftens the hair
    b) used with cold waves
    c) used on resistant hair types
    d) used to slow the processing action   _____

64. The main active ingredient in alkaline waves is:
    a) glyceryl monothioglycolate
    b) ammonium thioglycolate
    c) calcium hydroxide
    d) sodium hydroxide   _____

65. The pH range of alkaline waving lotions is generally:
    a) 7.0 to 7.6
    b) 8.0 to 8.6
    c) 9.0 to 9.6
    d) 10.0 to 10.6   _____

66. Characteristics of alkaline waving lotions include the following *except:*
    a) causes hair shaft shrinkage
    b) lifts the cuticle layer
    c) causes hair shaft swelling
    d) causes hair softening   _____

67. Benefits associated with alkaline perms include the following *except:*
    a) strong curl patterns
    b) room temperature processing
    c) faster processing time
    d) slower processing time   _____

68. Alkaline perms are generally used on hair that is considered to be:
    a) fragile
    b) resistant
    c) delicate
    d) color treated   _____

69. True acid waves have a pH range of:
    a) 2.5 to 7.0
    b) 3.5 to 7.5
    c) 4.5 to 7.0
    d) 7.0 to 8.5   _____

70. The primary reducing agent in true acid waves is:
    a) glyceryl monothioglycolate
    b) ammonium thioglycolate
    c) calcium hydroxide
    d) sodium hydroxide   _____

71. Characteristics associated with true acid waves include the following *except:*
    a) strong curl patterns
    b) less damaging than alkaline
    c) soft curl patterns
    d) may require dryer heat   _____

72. A perm product requiring the use a heat source to activate chemical reactions is called:
     a) exothermic   b) endothermic
     c) neutral   d) neither a, b, or c   _____

73. True acid perms should be used when permanent waving the following *except:*
     a) delicate hair   b) fragile hair
     c) color-treated hair   d) resistant hair   _____

74. Most acid-balanced waving lotions have a pH range of:
     a) 6.5 to 7.0   b) 4.5 to 7.5
     c) 7.8 to 8.2   d) 8.5 to 9.5   _____

75. The active ingredients in acid-balanced waving lotions are:
     a) AGT and GTMG   b) ATG and GMTG
     c) ATM and GTO   d) ATG and ATM   _____

76. Components of exothermic perms include the waving solution and the:
     a) activator and   b) activator and conditioner
        neutralizer
     c) neutralizer and   d) reducing agent and
        conditioner   neutralizer   _____

77. The active ingredients used in ammonia-free waves are:
     a) acids   b) hydroxides
     c) alkanolamines   d) oxides   _____

78. Characteristics of alkanolamines include the following *except:*
     a) slow evaporation   b) quick evaporation
     c) little to no odor   d) consistent pH level
                                   during processing   _____

79. Accidentally mixing the contents of the activator tube with the neutralizer will cause:
     a) violent chemical   b) neutralization
        reaction
     c) no chemical reaction   d) reduction   _____

80. The primary reducing agents used in thio-free waves are cysteamine or:
     a) alkanolamines   b) ammonium thioglycolate
     c) hydroxides   d) mercaptamine   _____

81. Characteristics of low-pH waves include the following *except:*
    a) sulfates, sulfites, and bisulfites
    b) do not produce a firm curl
    c) contain ATG
    d) usually marketed as body waves _____

82. The usual strengths of permanent-waving products include the following *except:*
    a) mild
    b) resistant
    c) normal
    d) super _____

83. Most prewraps are:
    a) leave-in conditioners
    b) neutralizers
    c) waving lotions
    d) activators _____

84. Most of the processing of a permanent wave takes place within:
    a) the first minute
    b) the first 5 minutes
    c) 5 to 10 minutes
    d) 10 to 20 minutes _____

85. Wave processing has reached its peak when it forms a firm:
    a) spiral shape
    b) letter S shape
    c) ridged shape
    d) letter C shape _____

86. Limp or weak wave formation is a sign of:
    a) overprocessing
    b) underprocessing
    c) curl formation
    d) optimum processing _____

87. Frizziness is an indication of
    a) overprocessing
    b) underprocessing
    c) curl formation
    d) optimum processing _____

88. To determine how the client's hair will react to the permanent-waving process, perform a:
    a) strand test
    b) color test
    c) patch test
    d) test curl _____

89. Two functions of a neutralizer are to deactivate remaining waving lotion in the hair and:
    a) to rebuild disulfide bonds
    b) to expand the cuticle
    c) to soften disulfide bonds
    d) to soften the cuticle _____

90. Permanently waved hair should be shampooed with:
    a) alkaline shampoos
    b) acid-balanced shampoos
    c) clarifying shampoos
    d) medicated shampoos _____

91. Three components of a soft curl perm are the waving lotion and the:
    a) neutralizer and water
    b) rearranger and conditioner
    c) rearranger and neutralizer
    d) booster and water
    _____

92. Chemically rearranging extremely curl hair into a straightened form is called:
    a) permanent waving
    b) chemical hair relaxing
    c) soft curl perming
    d) reformation curling
    _____

93. The basic products used in the chemical hair-relaxing process include the following except:
    a) waving lotion
    b) neutralizing shampoo
    c) relaxer cream
    d) conditioner
    _____

94. Two of the most common types of relaxers are the:
    a) acid and hydroxide
    b) thio and hydroxide
    c) acid and thio
    d) hydroxide and sodium
    _____

95. The type of relaxer product that requires a chemical neutralizing solution is the:
    a) acid relaxer
    b) sodium relaxer
    c) thio relaxer
    d) hydroxide relaxer
    _____

96. Characteristics of sodium hydroxide relaxers include the following except:
    a) known as lye relaxers
    b) pH range of 8.0 to 10.0
    c) pH range of 10 to 14
    d) oldest and most used
    _____

97. Characteristics of guanidine hydroxide relaxers include the following except:
    a) known as no-lye relaxers
    b) do not require mixing
    c) require mixing
    d) recommended for sensitive scalps
    _____

98. Characteristics of calcium hydroxide relaxers include the following except:
    a) very gentle on hair
    b) considered mild
    c) requires and activator
    d) work slowly on the hair
    _____

99. Base and no-base formulas refer to:
    a) thio relaxers
    b) reformation curls
    c) hydroxide relaxers
    d) soft curl perms
    _____

100. Texturizers and chemical blow-outs are used to:
    a) curl hair
    b) partially straighten hair
    c) straighten hair
    d) flat-iron hair
    _____

CHAPTER 19: HAIRCOLORING AND LIGHTENING

1. The science and art of changing the color of the hair is called:
   - a) hair lightening
   - b) hair dying
   - c) haircoloring
   - d) a chemical texture service _____

2. The partial or total removal of natural pigment or artificial color from the hair is called:
   - a) hair lightening
   - b) hair stripping
   - c) haircoloring
   - d) hair dying _____

3. Factors relevant to a haircoloring or lightening service include the following except:
   - a) texture and density
   - b) length and style
   - c) cuticle and cortex characteristics
   - d) porosity and natural color _____

4. Hair that accepts haircoloring products faster and permits darker saturation is considered:
   - a) nonporous
   - b) overporous
   - c) moderately porous
   - d) porous _____

5. Hair with a low porosity level has a cuticle that is:
   - a) tight
   - b) damaged
   - c) swollen
   - d) softened _____

6. Hair with a low porosity level is considered to be:
   - a) accepting of chemical penetration
   - b) perfect for chemical penetration
   - c) resistant to chemical penetration
   - d) neither a, b, nor c _____

7. Hair with a high porosity level has the following characteristics *except:*
   - a) has a lifted cuticle
   - b) able to resist color pigments
   - c) may take color quickly
   - d) may be unable to hold color _____

8. Natural hair color ranges from black to:
   - a) dark blond
   - b) lightest blond
   - c) pale blond
   - d) yellow-blond _____

9. The ratio of eumelanin to pheomelanin helps to determine:
   - a) hair density
   - b) hair texture
   - c) hair elasticity
   - d) natural hair color _____

10. The pigment that lies under the natural hair color is called:
   a) base pigment
   b) base melanin
   c) contributing pigment
   d) undertone _____

11. Color is a form of visible:
   a) energy
   b) light energy
   c) reflection
   d) deflection _____

12. The mixing of dyes and pigment to make other colors is regulated by the:
   a) laws of color
   b) artist's concepts
   c) laws of haircoloring
   d) availability of pigments _____

13. Primary colors include the following *except:*
   a) red
   b) yellow
   c) green
   d) blue _____

14. Secondary colors include the following *except:*
   a) red
   b) green
   c) orange
   d) violet _____

15. Colors with a predominance of blue are considered:
   a) warm colors
   b) cool-toned
   c) warm-toned
   d) neutral colors _____

16. Colors with a predominance of red are considered:
   a) neutral colors
   b) cool-toned
   c) warm-toned
   d) cool colors _____

17. Characteristics of the color blue include the following *except:*
   a) darkest primary color
   b) the only cool primary color
   c) ability to create depth and darkness to other colors
   d) the only neutral primary color _____

18. Characteristics of the color red include the following *except:*
   a) lightest primary color
   b) lightens blue-based colors
   c) medium primary color
   d) darkens yellow colors _____

19. Characteristics of the color yellow include the following *except:*
   a) is the lightest primary color
   b) lightens blue-based colors
   c) lightens red colors
   d) darkens orange colors _____

20. Mixing equal amounts of two primary colors will create:
    a) complementary colors b) secondary colors
    c) a or b   d) neither a nor b   _____

21. Mixing equal amounts of one primary color with one of
    its secondary colors creates a:
    a) new secondary color   b) quaternary color
    c) tertiary color   d) dark color   _____

22. Orange, green, and violet are examples of:
    a) primary colors   b) secondary colors
    c) tertiary colors   d) quaternary colors   _____

23. Yellow-green, blue-green, blue-violet, red-violet, red-
    orange, and yellow-orange are:
    a) primary colors   b) secondary colors
    c) tertiary colors   d) quaternary colors   _____

24. Two colors situated directly across from each other on
    the color wheel are called:
    a) complementary colors b) secondary colors
    c) primary colors   d) tertiary colors   _____

25. When two complementary colors are mixed together in
    equal amounts, they:
    a) brighten each other   b) neutralize each other
    c) darken each other   d) lighten each other   _____

26. The complementary color of blue is:
    a) red   b) orange
    c) green   d) violet   _____

27. The complementary color of red is:
    a) yellow   b) blue
    c) green   d) violet   _____

28. The complementary color of yellow is:
    a) red   b) blue
    c) green   d) violet   _____

29. Two types of colors that are composed of a primary and
    a secondary color are tertiary and:
    a) complementary   b) quaternary
    c) white   d) basic colors   _____

30. The basic name of a color is its tone or:
    a) level   b) place on the color wheel
    c) saturation   d) hue   _____

31. The terms associated with yellow, red, and orange colors include the following *except:*
    a) highlighting colors   b) cool colors
    c) warm colors   d) brightening colors   _____

32. The terms associated with green, blue, and violet colors include the following *except:*
    a) drab colors   b) cool colors
    c) warm colors   d) ashy colors   _____

33. The degree of lightness or darkness of a color is indicated by its:
    a) intensity   b) level
    c) tone   d) hue   _____

34. The level system is crucial to the following *except:*
    a) brand name color choice   b) matching colors
    c) formulating colors   d) correcting colors   _____

35. The degree of concentration or amount of pigment in a color is known as its:
    a) intensity or saturation   b) level
    c) tone   d) hue   _____

36. The predominant tone of a color is called its:
    a) hue   b) highlight
    c) base color   d) level   _____

37. The first step in performing a haircolor service is to identify the:
    a) color to use   b) natural level of the hair
    c) product to use   d) the desired color   _____

38. The four classifications of haircoloring products include temporary and the following *except:*
    a) semipermanent   b) permanent
    c) demipermanent   d) temporary semipermanent

39. Temporary haircolor products are a type of:
    a) oxidation color   b) penetrating color
    c) nonoxidation color   d) self-penetrating color   _____

40. Temporary haircolor lasts from:
    a) shampoo to shampoo   b) one to two shampoos
    c) two to four shampoos   d) four to six shampoos   _____

41. Characteristics of temporary color products include the following *except:*
    a) acidic chemical composition
    b) has a pH range of 2.0 to 4.5
    c) produce subtle color change
    d) penetrates to the cortex _____

42. Examples of temporary color products include the following *except:*
    a) henna
    b) color-enhancing shampoos
    c) instant and concentrated color rinses
    d) color crayons _____

43. Traditional semipermanent haircoloring products are a type of:
    a) oxidation color
    b) deep penetrating color
    c) nonoxidation color
    d) nonpenetrating color _____

44. Characteristics of semipermanent color products include the following *except:*
    a) mildly alkaline
    b) has a pH range of 7.0 to 9.0
    c) create only physical change
    d) slightly penetrates the cortex _____

45. Semipermanent haircolor lasts from:
    a) shampoo to shampoo
    b) six to eight shampoos
    c) two to four shampoos
    d) four to six shampoos _____

46. Semipermanent haircolor products require a:
    a) acid test
    b) elasticity test
    c) strand test
    d) patch test _____

47. Demipermanent haircoloring products are a type of:
    a) oxidation color
    b) progressive color
    c) nonoxidation color
    d) self-penetrating color _____

48. Characteristics of demiermanent color products include the following *except:*
    a) require a developer
    b) used directly from the bottle
    c) deposits color without lifting
    d) lasts longer than semipermanent color _____

49. Demipermanent haircolor products require a:
    a) porosity test
    b) predisposition test
    c) strand test
    d) elasticity test _____

50. A haircolor product that can lighten and deposit color in one process is a:
    a) temporary color   b) semipermanent color
    c) demipermanent color   d) permanent color   _____

51. Permanent haircoloring products are a type of:
    a) oxidation color   b) progressive color
    c) nonoxidation color   d) self-penetrating color   _____

52. Characteristics of permanent haircolor products include the following *except:*
    a) mixed with   b) do not need retouch
       hydrogen peroxide   applications
    c) deposit and lift   d) are penetrating tints   _____

53. The pH range of permanent haircolor products is:
    a) 7.0 to 8.5   b) 8.0 to 9.0
    c) 9.0 to 10.5   d) 11.0 to 14.0   _____

54. Permanent haircolor products require a:
    a) porosity test   b) patch test
    c) 9.0 to 10.5   d) elasticity test   _____

55. The best haircoloring product to use for covering gray hair is:
    a) temporary color   b) semipermanent color
    c) demipermanent color   d) permanent color   _____

56. Oxidation tints, vegetable tints, metallic dyes, and compound dyes are classifications of:
    a) temporary color   b) semipermanent color
    c) demipermanent color   d) permanent color   _____

57. Aniline derivative tints and penetrating tints are also known as:
    a) oxidation tints   b) neutralizing tints
    c) temporary tints   d) shampoo tints   _____

58. An example of a vegetable tint is:
    a) clay tint   b) synthetic plant tint
    c) henna   d) mineral tint   _____

58. Metallic or mineral dyes are marketed as:
    a) color enhancers   b) progressive colors
    c) a and b   d) neither a nor b   _____

60. Metallic or mineral dyes combined with a vegetable tint are called:
    a) combination dyes   b) compound dyes
    c) complex dyes   d) convoluted dyes   _____

61. A developer is a/an:
    a) coloring agent   b) toning agent
    c) oxidizing agent   d) stripping agent   _____

62. The primary oxidizing agent used in haircoloring is:
    a) hydrogen peroxide   b) ammonia
    c) water   d) dye remover   _____

63. When used as a developer, hydrogen peroxide has a pH range of:
    a) 1.0 to 2.0   b) 1.5 to 2.5
    c) 2.5 to 3.5   d) 3.5 to 4.0   _____

64. Measure of the potential oxidation of different hydrogen peroxide strengths is called:
    a) volume   b) decolorization
    c) lift   d) bleaching   _____

65. The higher the volume of hydrogen peroxide, the greater the:
    a) deposit action   b) neutralizing action
    c) lifting action   d) toning action   _____

66. Hydrogen peroxide is available in the following forms *except:*
    a) dry   b) gel
    c) cream   d) liquid   _____

67. Hydrogen peroxide formulations should not come into contact with:
    a) coloring products   b) hair
    c) skin   d) metal   _____

68. An oxidizer that is added to hydrogen peroxide to increase its chemical action is a/an:
    a) volume enhancer   b) inducer
    c) activator   d) deactivator   _____

69. A combination of a bleach formula and hydrogen peroxide produces:
    a) chemical heat   b) physical heat
    c) no change   d) static heat   _____

70. The actions of a lightener include the following *except:*
    a) decolorize natural   b) colorize natural
       hair pigment   hair pigment
    c) disperse natural   d) dissolve natural
       hair pigment   hair pigment   _____

71. For hair to lighten from the darkest color to the lightest, it must go through:
    a) four stages of lightening
    b) five stages of lightening
    c) six stages of lightening
    d) up to ten stages of lightening _____

72. Lighteners area available in the following forms *except:*
    a) mousses
    b) cream
    c) oil
    d) powder _____

73. Oil lighteners are usually mixtures of hydrogen peroxide with:
    a) hair oil tonic
    b) distilled water
    c) sulfonated oil
    d) alcohol _____

74. An oil lightener that removes pigment without adding color tone is a:
    a) gold oil lightener
    b) neutral oil lightener
    c) silver oil lightener
    d) drab oil lightener _____

75. The natural pigment that remains in the hair after lightening is called:
    a) foundation color
    b) underlying pigment
    c) base color
    d) underlying color _____

76. A haircoloring product that is applied to prelightened hair to achieve the desired shade is a:
    a) toner
    b) lightener
    c) dye remover
    d) dye solvent _____

77. Before application, toners require a:
    a) porosity test
    b) patch test
    c) strand test
    d) elasticity test _____

78. The removal of coloring agents is facilitated by:
    a) toners
    b) lighteners
    c) dye removers
    d) fillers _____

79. Haircoloring products with the ability to create a color base and equalize porosity are:
    a) toners
    b) lighteners
    c) dye removers
    d) fillers _____

80. Stain removers are prepared solutions that:
    a) remove tint from the skin
    b) remove lighteners from the hair
    c) remove color from the hair
    d) remove developer from color _____

81. A patch test is also known as a:
     a) color test   b) predisposition test
     c) disposition test   d) strand test   _____

82. Patch tests to determine allergies to aniline derivative tints should be performed:
     a) 1 to 2 hours   b) 4 to 6 hours
        before coloring   before coloring
     c) 24 to 48 hours   d) one week
        before coloring   before coloring   _____

83. A strand test is performed to determine the following *except:*
     a) reaction of hair   b) application method
        to product
     c) processing time   d) color results   _____

84. Equal parts of a prepared haircolor product and shampoo is called a:
     a) color rinse   b) tint back
     c) toner   d) soap cap   _____

85. The process that returns hair color to its natural shade is called a:
     a) color rinse   b) color remover
     c) tint back   d) soap cap   _____

86. The application of haircolor to hair that has not been previously colored is called a:
     a) virgin application   b) retouch application
     c) tint back application d) neither a, b, or c _____

87. A process that blends previously colored or lightened hair with new growth is a:
     a) virgin application   b) retouch application
     c) tint back application d) soap cap   _____

88. A process that lightens and colors the hair in a single application includes the following *except:*
     a) one-step coloring   b) single-application tinting
     c) one-step tinting   d) lightener and toner _____

89. Lightening and coloring actions are controlled independently during a:
     a) one-step coloring   b) double-application process
     c) one-step tinting   d) virgin application   _____

90. Lightening products that may be used on the scalp are:
    a) powder and oil lighteners
    b) cream and powder lighteners
    c) cream and oil lighteners
    d) any type of lightening product ____

91. Characteristics of powder lighteners include the following *except:*
    a) are on-the-scalp lighteners
    b) are off-the-scalp lighteners
    c) should not be used for retouch applications
    d) create blonding effects ____

92. The lightener generally used in a lightener retouch is a/an:
    a) powder lightener
    b) cream lightener
    c) oil lightener
    d) emollient lightener ____

93. Special-effects haircoloring and lightening include the following *except:*
    a) frosting
    b) streaking
    c) tipping
    d) scrunching ____

94. Special-effects application methods include the following *except:*
    a) foils
    b) wax paper
    c) cap
    d) free-form ____

95. Characteristics of gray hair include the following *except:*
    a) does not require analysis
    b) may require presoftening
    c) may be resistant to color
    d) is measured in percentages ____

96. Before tinting or lightening damaged hair, the hair should receive a:
    a) shampoo treatment
    b) haircut service
    c) reconditioning treatment
    d) clarifying treatment ____

97. Some over-the-counter haircoloring products may contain the following:
    a) coating dyes
    b) progressive dyes
    c) a or b
    d) neither a nor b ____

98. An aniline derivative tint should never be used for coloring:
    a) a mustache or beard
    b) retouch applications
    c) virgin hair
    d) gray hair ____

99. Characteristics of aniline derivatives include the following *except:*
    a) contain uncolored dye precursors
    b) contain colored dye precursors
    c) combine with hydrogen peroxide
    d) create permanent color molecules in the cortex _____

100. The process of treating resistant hair for better color penetration is called:
    a) pre-conditioning
    b) pre-expansion
    c) preparation
    d) pre-softening _____

CHAPTER 20: NAILS AND MANICURING

1. The main function of the nails is:
   a) cosmetic
   b) beautification
   c) protection
   d) absorption _____

2. The nail is composed of a translucent plate of:
   a) soft keratin
   b) hard keratin
   c) hard skin
   d) cartilage _____

3. Characteristics of the nail unit include the following parts *except* the:
   a) nail medulla
   b) nail bed
   c) nail root
   d) nail plate _____

4. The portion of the skin upon which the nail body rests is called the nail:
   a) nail folds
   b) nail bed
   c) nail root
   d) nail plate _____

5. The nail is formed and grows in the:
   a) nail folds
   b) nail bed
   c) nail root
   d) nail plate _____

6. The visible portion of the matrix bed is called the:
   a) launch
   b) lancet
   c) locator
   d) lunula _____

7. The visible portion of the nail is called the:
   a) nail bed
   b) nail plate
   c) nail root
   d) matrix _____

8. The nail body or nail plate extends from the:
   a) bed to the plate
   b) lunula to the bed
   c) root to the free edge
   d) lunula to the matrix _____

9. A crescent of overlapping epidermis around the base of the nail is called the:
   a) cuticle
   b) crust
   c) cortex
   d) callus _____

10. The extension of the cuticle that partly overlaps the lunula is the:
    a) eponychium
    b) melanonychia
    c) leukonychia
    d) hyponychium _____

11. The portion of the epidermis that lies under the free edge of the nail is the:
    a) eponychium
    b) melanonychia
    c) leukonychia
    d) hyponychium _____

12. Folds of normal skin that surround the nail plate are called the:
    a) nail folds
    b) nail walls
    c) a or b
    d) neither a nor b
    _____

13. The average nail growth per month is:
    a) $\frac{1}{8}$ inch
    b) $\frac{1}{4}$ inch
    c) $\frac{1}{2}$ inch
    d) 1 inch
    _____

14. The replacement of an injured nail is dependent on the health and condition of the:
    a) nail bed
    b) nail plate
    c) nail root
    d) matrix
    _____

15. The technical term applied to any deformity or disease of the nail is:
    a) melanonychia
    b) onychosis
    c) eponychium
    d) leukonychia
    _____

16. When a blood clot forms under the nail plate, the result is a/an:
    a) furrowed nail
    b) eggshell nail
    c) bruised nail
    d) hangnail
    _____

17. Nails that are thin, white, and curved at the free edge are called:
    a) furrowed nails
    b) eggshell nails
    c) bruised nails
    d) hangnails
    _____

18. Long ridges that run either lengthwise or across the nail are called:
    a) corrugations
    b) furrows
    c) a or b
    d) neither a nor b
    _____

19. A condition in which white spots appear on the nail due to air bubbles or bruising is:
    a) melanonychia
    b) onychosis
    c) eponychium
    d) leukonychia
    _____

20. A darkening of the nail as a result of localized pigment within the matrix bed is called:
    a) melanonychia
    b) onychosis
    c) eponychium
    d) leukonychia
    _____

21. Atrophy, or the wasting away, of the nail is called:
    a) onychauxis
    b) onychosis
    c) onychatrophia
    d) onychocryptosis
    _____

22. An abnormally thick overgrowth of the nails is called:
    a) onychauxis   b) onychosis
    c) onychatrophia   d) onychocryptosis   _____

23. The technical term for ingrown nails is:
    a) onychauxis   b) onychosis
    c) onychatrophia   d) onychocryptosis   _____

24. The technical term for deformed, bitten nails is:
    a) onychophagy   b) pterygium
    c) onychorrhexis   d) onychia   _____

25. Onychorrhexis is the technical term for:
    a) ingrown nails   b) enlarged nail curvature
    c) brittle or split nails d) pus formation at   _____
                                 the matrix

26. Forward growth of the cuticle on the nail is called:
    a) onychophagy   b) pterygium
    c) onychorrhexis   d) onychia   _____

27. An inflammation of the matrix with the formation of
    pus is known as:
    a) onychophagy   b) pterygium
    c) onychorrhexis   d) onychia   _____

28. Periodic shedding of the nail is called:
    a) onychoptosis   b) pterygium
    c) onychorrhexis   d) paronychia   _____

29. A bacterial inflammation of the tissue around the nail is:
    a) onychoptosis   b) pterygium
    c) onychorrhexis   d) paronychia   _____

30. Onychomycosis, or tinea unguim, is commonly known as:
    a) hangnails   b) ringworm of the nails
    c) ingrown nails   d) nail mold   _____

31. The surface of a nail buffer is made of leather or:
    a) silk   b) sandpaper
    c) suede   d) chamois   _____

32. Metal manicuring implements should be sanitized in a/an:
    a) disinfectant   b) alcohol
    c) antiseptic   d) ultraviolet-ray cabinet   _____

33. A cream that is used to lubricate and soften dry cuticles and brittle nails is a:
    a) hand cream   b) cuticle solvent
    c) cuticle cream   d) matrix cream   _____

34. Types of polish applications include the following methods *except:*
    a) full coverage   b) partial tip
    c) free-edge   d) hairline tip   _____

35. The squoval nail shape is a combination of a:
    a) square and oval shape   b) round and pointed shape
    c) round and oval shape   d) oval and pointed shape   _____

36. The nail shape most men *will not* prefer is the:
    a) square shape   b) pointed shape
    c) round shape   d) squoval shape   _____

37. Performing a manicure at the barber's workstation is called a:
    a) barber's manicure   b) standard manicure
    c) chairside manicure   d) shop manicure   _____

38. Nail conditions that should be treated by a physician include the following *except:*
    a) onychophagy   b) onychocryptosis
    c) infected nails   d) tinea   _____

39. Characteristics of tinea unguium include the following *except:*
    a) being known as onychomycosis   b) yellowish streaks within nail
    c) whitish patches on nail surface   d) no itching   _____

40. A relaxing service that is incorporated into the manicure procedure is the:
    a) hand and arm massage   b) neck massage
    c) scalp massage   d) foot massage   _____

CHAPTER 21: BARBERSHOP MANAGEMENT

1. Examples of self-employment in the barbering profession include the following *except:*
   a) booth rental
   b) barbershop owner
   c) independent contractor
   d) salaried employee _____

2. Generally, characteristics of a booth rental agreement include the following *except:*
   a) a barber chair is rented
   b) owner pays benefits
   c) tenant manages own clientele
   d) tenant is responsible for own taxes and supplies _____

3. Business operating expenses are also known as:
   a) overhead
   b) accounts receivables
   c) credits
   d) tax rebates _____

4. Some advantages to booth rental include the following *except:*
   a) low start-up investment
   b) self-employment
   c) need an established clientele
   d) being one's own boss _____

5. Booth rental necessitates that detailed and accurate records be kept for state and federal:
   a) labor inventories
   b) health plans
   c) income tax purposes
   d) property taxes _____

6. Barbershop management is primarily associated with production, daily operations, and:
   a) advertising
   b) bookkeeping
   c) marketing
   d) the people working in the shop _____

7. Characteristics of a sole-proprietor ownership include the following *except:*
   a) owner makes all decisions
   b) limited owner liability
   c) owner receives all profits
   d) owner is boss _____

8. Characteristics of a partnership arrangement include the following *except:*
   a) more available capital
   b) combined abilities
   c) shared losses and gains
   d) one decision maker _____

9. When three or more individuals own a business, an alternative to a partnership is a/an:
   a) corporation
   b) employer status
   c) sole-proprietorship
   d) neither a, b, nor c

   _____

10. A business structure in which stockholders are not legally responsible for losses is a:
    a) partnership
    b) corporation
    c) sole-proprietorship
    d) franchise

    _____

11. A franchise ownership may utilize:
    a) name recognition
    b) expertise and knowledge
    c) existing business systems
    d) a, b, and c

    _____

12. Before a business is purchased, it should be cleared of any ownership obligations or:
    a) financial obligations
    b) equipment
    c) signage
    d) fixtures and furnishings

    _____

13. A purchase agreement should include the following except:
    a) sales agreement
    b) inventory list
    c) a property lien
    d) financial disclosures

    _____

14. When planning to open a barbershop, the most important consideration is the selection of:
    a) depreciation
    b) social security
    c) a location
    d) advertising

    _____

15. A good location for a barbershop is near:
    a) other active businesses
    b) walk-by traffic
    c) drive-by traffic
    d) a, b, and c

    _____

16. A written description of the proposed business is called a/an:
    a) financial plan
    b) business plan
    c) design plan
    d) outlay plan

    _____

17. The working capital for a new business should be sufficient to cover expenses for at least:
    a) one year
    b) six months
    c) one quarter
    d) two years

    _____

18. The number one reason that businesses fail is due to:
    a) overcapitalization
    b) expertise
    c) undercapitalization
    d) business savvy

19. Local regulations *may* include the following *except:*
    a) building codes
    b) workers' compensation
    c) zoning laws
    d) occupational or
       business license   _____

20. State laws govern the following *except:*
    a) zoning laws
    b) professional licenses
    c) sales taxes
    d) workers' compensation   _____

21. Federal laws govern the following *except*:
    a) income tax
    b) social security
    c) local zoning laws
    d) OSHA safety and
       health standards   _____

22. Malpractice, premises liability, and fire refer to types of:
    a) compensation
    b) insurance
    c) taxes
    d) benefits   _____

23. A floor plan formalizes the barbershop:
    a) flooring choice
    b) lighting
    c) layout
    d) electrical requirements   _____

24. Activities that attract attention to the barbershop are considered to be forms of:
    a) advertising
    b) marketing
    c) goodwill
    d) a or b   _____

25. A document that protects a tenant from unexpected increases in rent is called a/an:
    a) insurance policy
    b) mortgage
    c) compensation policy
    d) lease   _____

26. Business success depends on effective, efficient management and the following *except:*
    a) noncompetitive
       services pricing
    b) sufficient investment
       capital
    c) trained personnel
    d) quality customer service   _____

27. Some contributing causes to business failure include the following *except:*
    a) high operational
       costs
    b) ideal location
    c) lack of business
       experience
    d) careless bookkeeping   _____

28. Rent, utilities, salaries, advertising, supplies, equipment, and repairs are classified as:
    a) expenses
    b) overhead
    c) operating costs
    d) a, b, or c   _____

29. To maintain accurate records that are processed in a timely manner, retain the services of a/an:
   a) lawyer   b) account
   c) manager   d) secretary   _____

30. The difference between total income and total expenses is the:
   a) accounts receivable   b) debits
   c) taxable income   d) net profit   _____

31. To keep expenditures on track, the business owner should maintain and utilize a/an:
   a) operating budget   b) checking account
   c) savings account   d) invoicing system   _____

32. The progress of a business can be evaluated by utilizing and maintaining:
   a) good employees   b) a lawyer
   c) summary sheets   d) an accountant   _____

33. Daily sales slips, appointment books, and petty cash receipts should be kept for at least:
   a) one week   b) one month
   c) one fiscal quarter   d) one year   _____

34. Payroll records, canceled checks, and monthly and yearly records are usually held for:
   a) three years   b) five years
   c) seven years   d) ten years   _____

35. When interviewing a prospective employee, the owner should consider the following *except:*
   a) personality and image   b) ethnicity
   c) grooming   d) communication skills

36. Managing employees effectively should include the following *except:*
   a) being honest with employees   b) sharing information
   c) expecting the best of employees   d) ignoring the rules   _____

37. Depending on the layout and procedures of the barbershop, financial transactions with clients are usually handled at the:
   a) reception desk   b) local bank
   c) front door   d) online payment center   _____

38. Generally, services on the appointment page are sold in terms of:
    a) cost
    b) time
    c) overhead
    d) neither a, b, or c
    _____

39. A significant amount of barbershop business is handled:
    a) at the chair
    b) over the Internet
    c) over the telephone
    d) at the barber's station
    _____

40. A good telephone personality includes the following characteristics *except:*
    a) a monotone voice
    b) clear speech
    c) a pleasing tone of voice
    d) correct speech patterns
    _____

41. Responding to customer complaints must *not* be handled with:
    a) tact
    b) self-control
    c) courtesy
    d) impatience
    _____

42. Successful selling in the barbershop requires a clear understanding of:
    a) the client's needs and desires
    b) knowledge of services
    c) retail product knowledge
    d) a, b, and c
    _____

43. Characteristics of an effective selling approach should include the following *except:*
    a) subtlety
    b) sincerity
    c) high pressure
    d) friendliness
    _____

44. Clients usually consider the barber to be an expert in:
    a) local sports
    b) good grooming
    c) the stock market
    d) politics
    _____

45. To facilitate greater cutting precision and to maintain sanitation standards, the barber should:
    a) shampoo the client's hair
    b) rinse hair from the comb
    c) wipe down the workstation
    d) reuse a soiled towel
    _____

CHAPTER 22: THE JOB SEARCH

1. Participation in barbershop operations while in school benefits students in the following *except:*
   a) experience
   b) opportunity
   c) no testing licensure
   d) understanding
   _____

2. Preparation for employment as a barber includes the following practical applications *except:*
   a) goal setting
   b) résumé writing
   c) professional activities
   d) sports activities
   _____

3. A student's participation in professional activities is of value to future employers because it:
   a) demonstrates initiative
   b) may indicate leadership skills
   c) shows interest in the profession
   d) a, b, or c
   _____

4. Some personal characteristics that help to attain a job position include the following *except:*
   a) good attitude
   b) tardiness
   c) enthusiasm
   d) strong work ethics
   _____

5. A barber's earnings or wages may be paid through:
   a) booth rental revenues
   b) a guarantee plus commission
   c) a commission structure
   d) a, b, or c
   _____

6. A written summary of one's education, work experience, and achievements is called a/an:
   a) résumé
   b) job application
   c) art portfolio
   d) sales kit
   _____

7. A collection of photographs depicting one's ability to provide hair care services is called a/an:
   a) résumé
   b) portfolio
   c) art portfolio
   d) sales kit
   _____

8. Field research in barbering refers to:
   a) writing a history paper
   b) networking and contacts
   c) visiting barbershops
   d) b and c
   _____

9. A standard practice of many barbershop employers is for job applicants to:

    a) perform a haircut or service   b) take an HIV test

    c) take a written test   d) provide a list of potential clients   _____

10. Appropriate actions for interviewing include the following *except:*

    a) dress for success   b) bring a bottle of water

    c) be prompt   d) be courteous   _____

11. Questions that *may not* be asked during an interview include the following *except:*

    a) smoker or non-smoker status   b) citizenship status

    c) race, religion, or national origin   d) disabilities or physical traits   _____

12. Questions that *may* be asked during an interview include the following *except:*

    a) smoker or nonsmoker status   b) citizenship status

    c) age   d) date of birth   _____

CHAPTER 23: STATE BOARD PREPARATION AND LICENSING LAWS

1. The event that marks the *beginning* of a professional career as a barber is:
   a) finishing barber school
   b) working as a barber
   c) taking state board exams
   d) renewing a barber license _____

2. A successful outcome to state board examinations is under the control of the:
   a) test candidate
   b) barber instructors
   c) barber board members
   d) barber examiners _____

3. An important preparation for written exams is to know:
   a) how to perform a haircut
   b) how to shave
   c) basic theory concepts
   d) how to give a perm _____

4. Important preparation for practical exams include:
   a) practice
   b) candidate information review
   c) state barber board rules review
   d) a, b, and c _____

5. The *primary* objective of barber licensing laws is to:
   a) limit number of licenses
   b) protect the public
   c) raise state revenue
   d) protect barbers _____

6. Licensing examinations are designed to evaluate an applicant's:
   a) competency
   b) goals
   c) attitudes
   d) endurance _____

7. Barber license law should never be used to:
   a) test competency
   b) limit number of licenses
   c) protect the client
   d) discipline barbers _____

8. Barbers who violate regulatory laws may be disciplined by license revocation or:
   a) renewal
   b) extension
   c) suspension
   d) display _____

9. A barber's license may not be revoked without:
   a) refunding the license fee
   b) due process of law
   c) a practical demonstration
   d) a new examination _____

10. Barbers accused of violating regulatory laws must be granted a:
    a) reprieve   b) extension
    c) suspension   d) hearing   _____

11. A person who practices barbering under the direct control of a licensed barber is a/an:
    a) journeyman barber   b) apprentice barber
    c) barbering student   d) barber instructor   _____

12. Individuals who are appointed to administer barbering laws and regulations are:
    a) state board members   b) journeymen barbers
    c) apprentice barbers   d) master barbers   _____

13. In pursuance of its duty to administer barber law, the board is authorized to issue:
    a) law amendments   b) unlawful decrees
    c) rules and regulations d) a strike   _____

14. Barbers who violate regulatory laws may be cited for:
    a) overcharging   b) taxation
    c) disciplinary action   d) undercharging   _____

15. Practicing barbering for remuneration without a license is:
    a) good business   b) unlawful
    c) basic compliance   d) contempt of court   _____

16. Barber license law requires that barber license applicants be:
    a) a U.S. citizen   b) over 21 years old
    c) at least 5 feet tall d) of good moral character   _____

17. A barber whose license has been revoked or suspended has the right to
    a) apply for a new   b) retake the examination
       license
    c) appeal to the courts d) disregard board orders   _____

18. A person convicted of a violation of barber law is guilty of a:
    a) misdemeanor   b) felony
    c) breach of contract   d) violation   _____

19. Barbershops are inspected periodically to ensure sanitation and:
    a) financial compliance b) signage compliance
    c) licensure compliance d) number of barbers
                                compliance   _____

20. The failure to display a license in a barbershop constitutes a:
    a) felony
    b) violation
    c) criminal act
    d) fraud
    _____

21. A barber's license that has been suspended or revoked must be:
    a) destroyed immediately
    b) surrendered to the board
    c) displayed in the shop
    d) subjected to a fine
    _____

22. A barber's license may be suspended, revoked, or denied if the barber is found guilty of:
    a) unauthorized leave of absence
    b) domestic difficulties
    c) motor vehicle violations
    d) gross malpractice
    _____

23. The responsibility of posting required documents and licenses in the barbershop rests with the:
    a) barbershop owner
    b) barber apprentice
    c) barber inspector
    d) board member
    _____

24. State barber boards regulate the following *except:*
    a) educational requirements
    b) haircut pricing
    c) testing and licensing
    d) inspections and investigations
    _____

25. Generally, persons who are legally exempt from barber law provisions are:
    a) nurses and doctors
    b) cosmetologists
    c) military personnel
    d) a, b, and c
    _____

Part II: Sample State Board Examinations

Directions: Read each statement carefully. Choose the word or phrase that most correctly completes the meaning of the statement and write the corresponding letter in the blank provided.

SAMPLE STATE BOARD EXAMINATION TEST 1

1. The word *barber* is derived from the Latin word *barba* meaning:
   - a) to cut
   - b) beard
   - c) shave
   - d) hairdresser   _____

2. Barber-surgeons participated in the practice of:
   - a) bloodletting
   - b) teeth pulling
   - c) surgery
   - d) a, b, and c   _____

3. In 1893, A. B. Moler established America's first barber:
   - a) trade journal
   - b) association
   - c) school
   - d) license   _____

4. State barber boards are primarily interested in maintaining high standards of:
   - a) appliances
   - b) tools
   - c) products
   - d) competency   _____

5. One key function of state barber boards is to protect the health, safety, and welfare of the:
   - a) profession
   - b) barbers
   - c) public
   - d) board members   _____

6. Personality, personal hygiene, and attitude are all aspects of an individual's:
   - a) grooming
   - b) barbering skills
   - c) professional image
   - d) health   _____

7. Proper behavior and business dealings with employers, clients, and coworkers is called:
   a) professional technique b) professional ethics
   c) career guidance   d) behavioral characteristics _____

8. Pathogenic bacteria produce:
   a) health   b) disease
   c) antitoxins   d) beneficial effects _____

9. Pus-forming organisms that grow in clusters and cause abscesses, pustules, pimples, and boils are:
   a) streptococci bacteria b) staphylococci bacteria
   c) diplococci bacteria   d) spirilla bacteria _____

10. Ringworm is caused by a/an:
    a) animal parasite   b) poison ivy
    c) bacterial parasite   d) plant parasite _____

11. Pediculosis is caused by:
    a) the itch mite   b) the body or head louse
    c) scabies   d) ringworm _____

12. The virus that causes AIDS is:
    a) HIB   b) HIV
    c) ARC   d) STD _____

13. The most likely manner in which HIV may be transmitted in the barbershop is by:
    a) shaking hands with   b) blood-to-blood contact
       an infected person   with an infected person
    c) using a soiled   d) using a sanitized
       headrest   comb _____

14. The removal of pathogens from tools and surfaces is known as:
    a) decontamination   b) contamination
    c) sepsis   d) cleaning _____

15. The process of thoroughly cleaning a tool or surface to its optimum level of decontamination in the barbershop is known as:
    a) sterilization   b) sanitizer
    c) disinfectant   d) disinfection or sanitation _____

16. State barber boards and health departments require only:
    a) sterilization   b) sanitation
       procedures   procedures
    c) disinfection   d) disinfection and
       procedures   sanitation procedures _____

17. A disinfectant that contains the properties of a bactericide, fungicide, pseudomonacide, virucide, and tuberculocide is considered to be a/an:
    a) minimal disinfectant
    b) hospital-level disinfectant
    c) deodorizer
    d) antiseptic _____

18. Antiseptics may be used on:
    a) the skin
    b) cutting implements
    c) dirty floors
    d) brushes and combs _____

19. For effective sanitization, the minimum strength of a quats solution used to sanitize implements is:
    a) 10%
    b) 1:2000
    c) 1:1000
    d) 20% _____

20. A wet sanitizer should contain:
    a) a disinfectant solution
    b) 30% alcohol
    c) an antiseptic solution
    d) 2% formalin _____

21. The Occupational Safety and Health Administration (OSHA) regulates and enforces safety and health in the workplace by:
    a) setting safety standards
    b) selling safe products
    c) causing worker injury
    d) importing products _____

22. Keep clean towels:
    a) near dirty towels
    b) in a clean, open cabinet
    c) in a clean, closed cabinet
    d) on a nearby shelf _____

23. Barbers should wash their hands:
    a) in the morning
    b) when they get dirty
    c) morning and afternoon
    d) before and after serving each client _____

24. Implements must be cleaned prior to immersion in a disinfectant solution to:
    a) avoid solution contamination
    b) comply with state board rules
    c) comply with sanitation procedures
    d) a, b, and c _____

25. When a blood spill occurs, employ:
    a) a doctor
    b) safety precautions
    c) universal precautions
    d) decontamination _____

26. Cream should be removed from jars with:
     a) the end of a used   b) tips of fingers
        towel
     c) a clean spatula   d) a comedone extractor   _____

27. Hair or other waste materials on the floor of a
    barbershop should be:
     a) swept into   b) placed in a
        a corner   closed container
     c) placed in a   d) swept up at the
        garbage can   end of the day   _____

28. Small nicks or cuts should be cleansed and
    treated with:
     a) a band aid   b) soap and water
     c) styptic powder   d) styptic pencil   _____

29. The most desirable type of hair comb is made of:
     a) plastic   b) metal
     c) bone   d) hard rubber   _____

30. The French type of haircutting shears:
     a) has no finger brace   b) has one finger brace
     c) has two finger braces d) does not have a shank   _____

31. When holding haircutting shears properly, the barber
    places the thumb in the thumb grip of the:
     a) shank   b) still blade
     c) moving blade   d) finger grip   _____

32. Electric clippers are driven by rotary motor, magnetic
    motor, or:
     a) circular motor   b) pivot motor
     c) vibratory motor   d) motor action   _____

33. Headrest covers must be changed:
     a) for each client   b) whenever they get soiled
     c) for every three clients d) for every other client   _____

34. The size clipper blade that produces the shortest cut is:
     a) size 0   b) size 0000
     c) size 000   d) size 00   _____

35. The first step in sanitizing clippers and trimmers is to:
     a) brush off hair   b) immerse blades in
        particles   blade wash
     c) immerse blades   d) spray with
        in water   disinfectant   _____

36. A straight razor is properly balanced when:
    a) the weight of the head equals that of the tang
    b) the weight of the blade equals that of the handle
    c) the weight of the blade does not equal that of the handle
    d) it does not pivot
    _____

37. The size of a razor is measured by the blade's:
    a) length
    b) thickness
    c) sharpness
    d) length and width
    _____

38. Honing and stropping are necessary for such implements as:
    a) haircutting shears
    b) thinning shears
    c) conventional straight razors
    d) hair clippers
    _____

39. The purpose of a hone is to:
    a) grind the razor's edge
    b) smooth the razor's edge
    c) polish the razor's edge
    d) align the razor's cutting teeth
    _____

40. The purpose of a strop is to:
    a) grind the razor's edge
    b) smooth the razor's edge
    c) polish the razor's edge
    d) impart a cutting edge to the razor
    _____

41. The shell or Russian shell strop is created from:
    a) the rump area of the horse
    b) cowhide
    c) synthetic materials
    d) canvas
    _____

42. The least acceptable method of removing loose hair after a haircut is the:
    a) small electric vacuum
    b) clean, folded towel
    c) unsanitized neck duster
    d) paper neck strips
    _____

43. An implement used to press out blackheads is a/an:
    a) tweezers
    b) comedone extractor
    c) electric hair vacuum
    d) electric latherizer
    _____

44. The basic units of the structure and function of all living things are:
    a) nuclei
    b) cells
    c) centrosome
    d) living matter
    _____

45. The skull consists of eight cranial bones and:
    a) 8 facial bones
    b) 10 facial bones
    c) 12 facial bones
    d) 14 facial bones
    _____

46. The occipital bone forms the back and base of the:
    a) neck   b) cranium
    c) upper jaw   d) forehead   _____

47. The more fixed attachment of a muscle to the bone is called the:
    a) origin   b) insertion
    c) joint   d) ligament   _____

48. Muscle tissue may be stimulated by massage, electric current, and:
    a) heat and light rays   b) nerve impulses and
                               chemicals
    c) moist heat   d) a, b, and c   _____

49. The largest and most complex nerve tissue in the body is/are the:
    a) lungs   b) spleen
    c) brain   d) heart   _____

50. Nerves may be stimulated by high-frequency current, moist heat, and:
    a) chemicals   b) light and heat rays
    c) massage   d) a, b, and c   _____

51. The main sources of blood to the head, face, and neck are supplied by the
    a) jugular veins   b) common carotid arteries
    c) arteries   d) veins   _____

52. The skin and its appendages make up the:
    a) integumentary system b) endocrine system
    c) circulatory system   d) capillary system   _____

53. The four types of matter are solids, liquids, gases, and:
    a) solutions   b) mixtures
    c) plasmas   d) compounds   _____

54. The liquid that is considered to be a universal solvent is:
    a) alcohol   b) peroxide
    c) bleach   d) water   _____

55. The best type of water to use in the barbershop is:
    a) distilled water   b) mineral water
    c) soft water   d) hard water   _____

56. The pH of a solution measures its degree of:
    a) softness or hardness   b) acidity or alkalinity
    c) heat or cold level   d) neutrality   _____

57. The pH range of hair and skin is:
    a) 3.5 to 4.5   b) 4.5 to 6.5
    c) 4.5 to 5.5   d) 5.5 to 6.5   _____

58. Acidic solutions will neutralize the effects of:
    a) alkaline solutions   b) salt solutions
    c) heat or cold conditions d) stress on the hair   _____

59. A mixture of two or more substances that is made
    by dissolving a solid, liquid, or gaseous substance in
    another substance is known as a/an:
    a) solution   b) ointment
    c) suspension   d) powder   _____

60. Cosmetic preparations that will cause the contraction of
    skin tissues are:
    a) fresheners   b) astringents
    c) facial toners   d) a, b, and c   _____

61. The basic purpose of a cold cream is to:
    a) eradicate wrinkles   b) cleanse the skin
    c) strengthen facial   d) reduce fat cells   _____
       muscles

62. Preparations that temporarily remove superfluous hair
    by dissolving it at the skin line are:
    a) depilatories   b) epilators
    c) razors   d) waxes   _____

63. Scalp lotions and ointments usually contain:
    a) surfactants   b) witch hazel
    c) alcohol   d) medicinal agents   _____

64. The primary ingredient in styptic powder or liquid is:
    a) talc   b) alum
    c) alcohol   d) witch hazel   _____

65. Witch hazel is a solution that acts as a/an:
    a) astringent   b) emulsion
    c) suspension   d) acid   _____

66. An electrical current flowing first in one direction
    and then in the opposite direction is called:
    a) direct current   b) tesla current
    c) alternating current d) galvanic current   _____

67. Electric clippers and hair dryers are examples of
    barbering tools that use:
    a) alternating current   b) converted current
    c) direct current   d) rectified current   _____

68. All electrical appliances used in the barbershop should be:
    a) Barber Board certified b) FDA certified
    c) UL certified   d) OSHA certified   _____

69. An applicator that directs electric current from the machine to the client's skin is a/an:
    a) conductor   b) modality
    c) electrode   d) massager   _____

70. The high-frequency current commonly used in the barbershop is the:
    a) d'Arsonval current   b) Oudin current
    c) sinusoidal current   d) tesla current   _____

71. For a stimulating effect, the high-frequency electrode is:
    a) slightly lifted from   b) in close contact with
       the skin   the skin
    c) held by the client   d) turned very low   _____

72. Ultraviolet rays produce:
    a) heat   b) germicidal reactions
    c) chemical reactions   d) b and c   _____

73. Ultraviolet rays are usually applied:
    a) 12 to 16 inches   b) 18 to 20 inches
       from the skin   from the skin
    c) 20 to 24 inches   d) 30 to 36 inches
       from the skin   from the skin   _____

74. The two main divisions of the skin are the epidermis and the:
    a) medulla   b) dermis
    c) cuticle   d) scarf skin   _____

75. The outer protective layer of the skin is called the scarf skin or the:
    a) dermis   b) adipose tissue
    c) epidermis   d) subcutaneous tissue   _____

76. The color of the skin is due to the amount of blood it contains and:
    a) keratin   b) moisture
    c) fat   d) melanin   _____

77. The stratum germinativum is the innermost layer of the:
    a) dermis   b) epidermis
    c) subcutaneous   d) corium   _____

154

78. The dermis is also known as the corium, cutis, derma, and:
    a) cuticle   b) false skin
    c) true skin   d) fatty tissue   _____

79. Subcutaneous tissue is also known as:
    a) muscle tissue   b) soft tissue
    c) adipose tissue   d) hard tissue   _____

80. The sebaceous glands are duct glands that secrete:
    a) melanin   b) sebum
    c) saliva   d) perspiration   _____

81. A structural change in the tissues caused by injury or disease is known as a:
    a) tumor   b) lesion
    c) cyst   d) fissure   _____

82. Examples of primary lesions include the following *except:*
    a) bulla, cyst, macule   b) vesicle, wheal
    c) papule, pustule,   d) scar, fissure, keloid   _____
       tubercle

83. Examples of secondary lesions include the following *except:*
    a) bulla, cyst, macule   b) scale, scab
    c) excoriation, crust   d) scar, fissure, keloid   _____

84. A skin wart is known as a:
    a) keloid   b) keratoma
    c) verruca   d) nevus   _____

85. The general term for an inflammatory condition of the skin is:
    a) trichology   b) dermatology
    c) histology   d) dermatitis   _____

86. Comedone is the technical name for a:
    a) whitehead   b) pimple
    c) blackhead   d) dry skin   _____

87. Acne is a disorder of the:
    a) sweat glands   b) oil glands
    c) intestinal glands   d) stomach glands   _____

88. An inflammatory skin disease that may be acute or chronic with dry or moist lesions is:
    a) eczema   b) seborrhea
    c) psoriasis   d) herpes simplex   _____

89. A recurring viral infection that produces fever blisters or cold sores is:
    a) eczema
    b) herpes simplex
    c) psoriasis
    d) dermatitis venenata
    _____

90. The most common and least severe type of skin cancer is:
    a) squamous cell carcinoma
    b) malignant melanoma
    c) basal cell carcinoma
    d) melanoma
    _____

91. Hair is chiefly composed of a horny substance called:
    a) hemoglobin
    b) melanin
    c) keratin
    d) calcium
    _____

92. That portion of the hair found beneath the skin surface is called the:
    a) hair root
    b) hair bulb
    c) hair shaft
    d) hair papilla
    _____

93. A small, cone-shaped elevation at the base of the hair follicle is called the:
    a) dermal papilla
    b) hair bulb
    c) hair shaft
    d) hair follicle
    _____

94. Glands that secrete sebum to the hair and scalp are called:
    a) sudoriferous glands
    b) follicle glands
    c) sebaceous glands
    d) excretion glands
    _____

95. The three main layers of the hair shaft are the:
    a) cuticle, cortex, and medulla
    b) follicle, root, and bulb
    c) root, bulb, and dermal papilla
    d) follicle, root, and papilla
    _____

96. That portion of the hair that provides strength, elasticity, and natural color is the:
    a) medulla
    b) hair shaft
    c) cortex
    d) cuticle
    _____

97. Chains of joined amino acids are known as:
    a) amino chains
    b) end chains
    c) chemical chains
    d) polypeptide chains
    _____

98. Hair grows an average of:
    a) $\frac{1}{4}$ inch per month
    b) $\frac{1}{2}$ inch per month
    c) $\frac{3}{4}$ inch per month
    d) 1 inch per month
    _____

99. The term used to indicate the number of individual hair strands per square inch of scalp area is:
    a) density
    b) porosity
    c) elasticity
    d) texture
    _____

100. The ability of the hair to absorb moisture determines its:
    a) level of density
    b) level of porosity
    c) level of elasticity
    d) variation in texture
    _____

101. Alopecia is the technical term for any abnormal type of:
    a) hair loss
    b) skin inflammation
    c) oil gland disorder
    d) sweat gland disorder
    _____

102. Common scalp disorders include dandruff, vegetable and animal parasitic infections, and:
    a) diplococcal infections
    b) streptococcal infections
    c) staphylococcal infections
    d) pediculosis infestations
    _____

103. Small, white scales appearing on the scalp and hair is a sign of:
    a) dermatitis
    b) eczema
    c) herpes simplex
    d) pityriasis
    _____

104. Ringworm of the scalp is the common name for:
    a) tinea
    b) tinea favosa
    c) tinea capitis
    d) tinea sycosis
    _____

105. All forms of tinea are:
    a) nontreatable
    b) contagious
    c) noncontagious
    d) treatable by the barber
    _____

106. Pediculosis and scabies are:
    a) nontreatable
    b) not contagious
    c) contagious infestations
    d) treatable by the barber
    _____

107. Inflammations of the follicle caused by bacteria or irritation may be signs of:
    a) folliculitis
    b) pseudofolliculitis barbae
    c) a or b
    d) neither a nor b
    _____

108. The main purpose of a shampoo is to:
    a) make hair easier to comb
    b) cleanse the hair and scalp
    c) treat alopecia areata
    d) soften the scalp
    _____

109. Solutions that soften, swell, or expand the cuticle scales usually have a/an:
    a) acidic pH level
    b) neutral pH level
    c) alkaline pH level
    d) harsh pH level

    _____

110. The portion of the shampoo molecule that attracts water and repels dirt is the:
    a) head
    b) middle
    c) belly
    d) tail

    _____

111. The type of shampoo that is very effective in reducing dandruff is the:
    a) green soap shampoo
    b) therapeutic medicated shampoo
    c) liquid dry shampoo
    d) egg shampoo

    _____

112. Rinses that are formulated to control minor dandruff and scalp conditions are:
    a) water rinses
    b) bluing rinses
    c) medicated rinses
    d) tonic rinses

    _____

113. A cosmetic solution that can stimulate the scalp, correct a scalp condition, or be used as a grooming aid is a:
    a) conditioner
    b) styling spray
    c) hair tonic
    d) scalp ointment

    _____

114. The purpose of a towel or neck strip between the drape and the client's skin is to:
    a) maintain sanitation standards
    b) conform to state barber laws
    c) prevent drape contact with client's skin
    d) a, b, and c

    _____

115. The two methods employed by barbers to perform a shampoo service are the:
    a) upright and reclined methods
    b) inclined and reclined methods
    c) tub and shower methods
    d) backward and reclined methods

    _____

116. Shampoo and scalp manipulations are performed with:
    a) the cushions of the fingertips
    b) fingernails
    c) rubber gloves
    d) disposable gloves

    _____

117. Scalp massage should be performed with:
    a) fast motion and no pressure
    b) slow motion and no pressure
    c) continuous, even motion and pressure
    d) fast motion and heavy pressure

    _____

118. Barbers are qualified to perform treatments for the following *except:*
    a) dry scalp
    b) oily scalp and hair
    c) dandruff
    d) parasitic or staphylococcus conditions
    _____

119. Scalp massage is beneficial because it stimulates the:
    a) salivary glands
    b) blood circulation
    c) pituitary gland
    d) thyroid gland
    _____

120. Conditions that may prohibit a facial massage include the following *except:*
    a) high blood pressure
    b) severe skin lesions
    c) skin inflammation
    d) normal skin
    _____

121. A point on the skin where pressure or stimulation will cause contraction of the muscle is a/an:
    a) motor point
    b) trigger point
    c) sensory point
    d) secretory point
    _____

122. Effleurage is used in massage for its:
    a) stimulating effects
    b) soothing and relaxing effects
    c) heating effects
    d) frictional effects
    _____

123. Facials performed in the barbershop are considered to be either:
    a) preventive or corrective
    b) corrective or medicinal
    c) preventive or medicinal
    d) corrective or therapeutic
    _____

124. The four skin types include dry, normal, combination, and:
    a) sensitive
    b) allergic
    c) irritated
    d) oily
    _____

125. When shaving a client, professional barbers use warm lather and a conventional:
    a) disposable safety razor
    b) straight razor
    c) safety razor
    d) electric razor
    _____

126. All of the following may cause ingrown hairs *except:*
    a) excessively close shaving
    b) shear cutting
    c) excessive pressure
    d) improper use of tweezers, razor, or trimmers
    _____

127. To achieve the best cutting stroke, the razor must glide over the surface at an angle:
    a) against the grain of the hair
    b) with the grain of the hair
    c) across the grain of the hair
    d) diagonal to the grain of the hair
    _____

128. When shaving, a gliding stroke directed toward the barber is used with the:
    a) freehand stroke
    b) backhand stroke
    c) cutting stroke
    d) reverse freehand stroke
    _____

129. Close shaving is the practice of shaving the beard:
    a) against or across the grain
    b) with the grain of the hair
    c) across the grain of the hair
    d) diagonal to the grain of the hair
    _____

130. Facial shapes are determined by the position and prominence of the:
    a) forehead
    b) nose
    c) chin
    d) facial bones
    _____

131. A tapered haircut is usually longer in the crown and top areas and:
    a) shorter at the nape
    b) uniform at the nape
    c) longer at the nape
    d) neither a, b, or c
    _____

132. The removal of excess bulk from the hair is called:
    a) slithering
    b) dethickening
    c) customizing
    d) thinning
    _____

133. When using the shear-over-comb technique, the hair is placed in position for cutting by:
    a) combing through it
    b) holding hair between the fingers
    c) brushing through the hair
    d) rolling the comb out
    _____

134. The standard clipper cutting techniques are the:
    a) freehand and backhand
    b) clipper-over-comb and freehand
    c) freehand and underhand
    d) clipper-over-comb and backhand
    _____

135. The type of cutting method that can help make resistant hair textures more manageable is:
    a) clipper cutting
    b) razor cutting
    c) shear cutting
    d) hair singeing
    _____

136. Razor cutting requires that the hair be:
    a) chemically processed b) clean and damp
    c) clean and dry   d) misted   _____

137. Shaving the sides of the neck and across the nape with a
    razor is called a/an:
    a) extra service   b) outline shave
    c) neck shave   d) hairline shave   _____

138. Hair replacement techniques include toupees or
    hairpieces and the following *except:*
    a) certain drugs   b) chemical processes
    c) surgical hair   d) scalp reduction
       transplantation   _____

139. Hairpieces made of human hair must be:
    a) shampooed and   b) dry cleaned
       conditioned
    c) washed with   d) cleaned with
       warm water   acetone   _____

140. Hairpieces may be cut and blended with shears or
    a/an:
    a) clipper   b) outliner
    c) razor   d) edger   _____

141. The process used to chemically restructure straight hair
    into a different wave pattern is:
    a) permanent waving   b) haircoloring
    c) reformation curls   d) hair relaxing   _____

142. A reformation curl is also known as the following *except:*
    a) chemical blow-out   b) Jheri curl
    c) soft-curl perm   d) a curl   _____

143. The process used to rearrange overcurly hair into a
    straightened hair form is known as:
    a) permanent wave   b) a curl
    c) reformation curl   d) chemical hair relaxing   _____

144. The two layers of the hair most affected by chemical
    texture services are the:
    a) cortex and medulla   b) cortex and cuticle
    c) medulla and cuticle d) cortex and hair root   _____

145. The partial or total removal of natural pigment or
    artificial color from the hair is called:
    a) hair lightening   b) hair stripping
    c) haircoloring   d) hair dying   _____

146. The four classifications of haircoloring products include temporary and the following *except:*
    a) semipermanent
    b) permanent
    c) demipermanent
    d) temporary semipermanent   _____

147. Temporary haircolor products are a type of:
    a) oxidation color
    b) penetrating color
    c) nonoxidation color
    d) self-penetrating color   _____

148. Characteristics of permanent haircolor products include the following *except:*
    a) mixed with hydrogen peroxide
    b) do not need retouch applications
    c) deposit and lift
    d) are penetrating tints   _____

149. A patch test that results in redness or inflammation indicates the presence of a/an:
    a) immunity
    b) allergy
    c) blister
    d) verruca   _____

150. The technical term applied to any deformity or disease of the nail is:
    a) onychosis
    b) melanonychia
    c) eponychium
    d) leukonychia   _____

SAMPLE STATE BOARD EXAMINATION TEST 2

1. The word *barber* is derived from the Latin word *barba* meaning:
   - a) to cut
   - b) beard
   - c) shave
   - d) hairdresser   _____

2. Barber-surgeons participated in the practice of:
   - a) bloodletting
   - b) teeth pulling
   - c) surgery
   - d) a, b, and c   _____

3. State barber boards are primarily interested in maintaining high standards of:
   - a) appliances
   - b) tools
   - c) products
   - d) competency   _____

4. One key function of state barber boards is to protect the health, safety, and welfare of the:
   - a) profession
   - b) barbers
   - c) public
   - d) board members   _____

5. Proper behavior and business dealings with employers, clients, and coworkers is called:
   - a) professional technique
   - b) professional ethics
   - c) career guidance
   - d) behavioral characteristics   _____

6. Pathogenic bacteria produce:
   - a) health
   - b) disease
   - c) antitoxins
   - d) beneficial effects   _____

7. Pus-forming organisms that grow in clusters and cause abscesses, pustules, pimples, and boils are:
   - a) staphylococci bacteria
   - b) streptococci bacteria
   - c) diplococci bacteria
   - d) spirilla bacteria   _____

8. Pustules and boils contain:
   - a) nonpathogenic organisms
   - b) pathogenic bacteria
   - c) sweat
   - d) ringworm   _____

9. During the active stage, bacteria:
   - a) vegetate
   - b) lie dormant
   - c) grow and reproduce
   - d) form spores   _____

10. Ringworm is caused by a/an:
    - a) animal parasite
    - b) poison ivy
    - c) bacterial parasite
    - d) plant parasite   _____

11. Pediculosis is caused by:
    - a) the itch mite
    - b) the body or head louse
    - c) scabies
    - d) ringworm   _____

12. The virus that causes AIDS is:
    - a) HIV
    - b) HIB
    - c) ARC
    - d) STD   _____

13. The most likely manner in which HIV may be transmitted in the barbershop is by:
    - a) shaking hands with an infected person
    - b) blood-to-blood contact with an infected person
    - c) using a soiled headrest
    - d) using a sanitized comb   _____

14. The removal of pathogens from tools and surfaces is known as:
    - a) decontamination
    - b) contamination
    - c) sepsis
    - d) cleaning   _____

15. The process of thoroughly cleaning a tool or surface to its optimum level of decontamination in the barbershop is known as:
    - a) sterilization
    - b) sanitizer
    - c) disinfectant
    - d) disinfection or sanitation   _____

16. State barber boards and health departments require only:
    - a) sterilization procedures
    - b) sanitation procedures
    - c) disinfection procedures
    - d) disinfection and sanitation procedures   _____

17. A disinfectant that contains the properties of a bactericide, fungicide, pseudomonacide, virucide, and tuberculocide is considered to be a/an:
    - a) minimal disinfectant
    - b) hospital- level disinfectant
    - c) deodorizer
    - d) antiseptic   _____

18. Antiseptics may be used on:
    - a) the skin
    - b) cutting implements
    - c) dirty floors
    - d) brushes and combs   _____

19. For effective sanitization, the minimum strength of a quat solution used to sanitize implements is:
    - a) 10%
    - b) 1:2000
    - c) 1:1000
    - d) 20%   _____

20. A wet sanitizer should contain:
    a) a disinfectant   b) 30% alcohol
       solution
    c) an antiseptic solution   d) 2% formalin   _____

21. The Occupational Safety and Health Administration
    (OSHA) regulates and enforces safety and health in the
    workplace by:
    a) setting safety   b) selling safe products
       standards
    c) causing worker injury   d) importing products   _____

22. Keep clean towels:
    a) near dirty towels   b) in a clean, open cabinet
    c) in a clean, closed   d) on a nearby shelf   _____
       cabinet

23. Barbers should wash their hands:
    a) in the morning   b) when they get dirty
    c) morning and   d) before and after serving
       afternoon   each client   _____

24. Implements must be cleaned prior to immersion in a
    disinfectant solution to:
    a) avoid solution   b) comply with
       contamination   state board rules
    c) comply with   d) a, b, and c
       sanitation procedures   _____

25. When a blood spill occurs, employ:
    a) a doctor   b) safety precautions
    c) universal precautions   d) decontamination   _____

26. Cream should be removed from jars with:
    a) the end of a used   b) tips of fingers
       towel
    c) a clean spatula   d) a comedone extractor   _____

27. Hair or other waste materials on the floor of a
    barbershop should be:
    a) swept into a corner   b) placed in a closed container
    c) placed in a   d) swept up at the end of
       garbage can   the day   _____

28. Small nicks or cuts should be cleansed and treated with:
    a) a band aid   b) soap and water
    c) styptic powder   d) styptic pencil   _____

29. The most desirable type of hair comb is made of:
    a) plastic   b) metal
    c) bone   d) hard rubber   _____

30. The French type of haircutting shears:
    a) has no finger brace   b) has one finger brace
    c) has two finger braces d) does not have a shank   _____

31. When holding haircutting shears properly, the barber
    places the thumb in the thumb grip of the:
    a) shank   b) still blade
    c) moving blade   d) finger grip   _____

32. Electric clippers are driven by rotary motor, magnetic
    motor, or:
    a) circular motor   b) pivot motor
    c) vibratory motor   d) motor action   _____

33. Headrest covers must be changed:
    a) for each client   b) whenever they get soiled
    c) for every three clients d) for every other client _____

34. The clipper blade size that leaves the hair the longest is:
    a) size 1   b) size 2
    c) size $1\frac{1}{2}$ d) size 3   _____

35. The first step in sanitizing clippers and trimmers is to:
    a) brush off   b) immerse blades
       hair particles   in blade wash
    c) immerse blades   d) spray with
       in water   disinfectant   _____

36. The grind of a razor refers to the shape of the:
    a) tang   b) heel
    c) blade   d) handle   _____

37. The size of a razor refers is measured by the blade's:
    a) length   b) thickness
    c) sharpness   d) length and width   _____

38. A crocus finish on the blade of a razor is also known as:
    a) nickel-plated finish   b) silver-plated finish
    c) plain steel finish   d) polished-steel finish   _____

39. The purpose of a hone is to:
    a) grind the   b) smooth the
       razor's edge   razor's edge
    c) polish the   d) align the razor's
       razor's edge   cutting teeth   _____

166

40. The purpose of a strop is to:
    a) grind the
       razor's edge
    b) smooth the
       razor's edge
    c) polish the
       razor's edge
    d) impart a cutting edge
       to the razor   _____

41. The shell or Russian shell strop is created from:
    a) the rump area of
       the horse
    b) cowhide
    c) synthetic materials
    d) canvas   _____

42. The direction used in razor stropping is:
    a) the same as that
       used in honing
    b) in a counter-
       clockwise direction
    c) the reverse of that
       used in honing
    d) in a clockwise
       direction   _____

43. An implement used to press out blackheads is a/an:
    a) tweezers
    b) comedone extractor
    c) electric hair vacuum
    d) electric latherizer   _____

44. The least acceptable method of removing loose hair
    after a haircut is the:
    a) small electric
       vacuum
    b) clean towel,
       properly folded
    c) unsanitized
       neck duster
    d) paper neck strips   _____

45. The skull consists of eight cranial bones and:
    a) 8 facial bones
    b) 10 facial bones
    c) 12 facial bones
    d) 14 facial bones   _____

46. The occipital bone forms the back and base of the:
    a) neck
    b) cranium
    c) upper jaw
    d) forehead   _____

47. The least fixed attachment of a muscle to the bone is
    called the:
    a) origin
    b) insertion
    c) joint
    d) ligament   _____

48. Muscle tissue may be stimulated by massage, electric
    current, and:
    a) heat and light rays
       chemicals
    b) nerve impulses and
    c) moist heat
    d) a, b, and c   _____

49. The parietal bones form the top and sides of the:
    a) face
    b) cranium
    c) cheeks
    d) neck   _____

50. Nerves may be stimulated by high-frequency current, moist heat, and:
    a) chemicals
    b) light and heat rays
    c) massage
    d) a, b, and c
    _____

51. The main sources of blood to the head, face, and neck are supplied by the
    a) jugular veins
    b) common carotid arteries
    c) arteries
    d) veins
    _____

52. The skin and its appendages make up the:
    a) integumentary system
    b) endocrine system
    c) circulatory system
    d) capillary system
    _____

53. Twelve pairs of cranial nerves branch out from the brain and reach parts of the:
    a) arms and hands
    b) legs and feet
    c) abdomen and back
    d) head, face, and neck
    _____

54. The liquid that is considered to be a universal solvent is:
    a) alcohol
    b) peroxide
    c) bleach
    d) water
    _____

55. The best type of water to use in the barbershop is:
    a) distilled water
    b) mineral water
    c) soft water
    d) hard water
    _____

56. The pH of a solution measures its degree of:
    a) softness or hardness
    b) acidity or alkalinity
    c) heat or cold level
    d) neutrality
    _____

57. The pH range of hair and skin is:
    a) 3.5 to 4.5
    b) 4.5 to 6.5
    c) 4.5 to 5.5
    d) 5.5 to 6.5
    _____

58. An example of a suspension is:
    a) a quat solution
    b) hair oil tonic
    c) witch hazel
    d) shampoo
    _____

59. A mixture of two or more substances that is made by dissolving a solid, liquid, or gaseous substance in another substance is known as a/an:
    a) solution
    b) ointment
    c) suspension
    d) powder
    _____

60. Cosmetic preparations that will cause the contraction of skin tissues are:
    a) fresheners
    b) astringents
    c) facial toners
    d) a, b, and c
    _____

61. The basic purpose of a cold cream is to:
    a) eradicate wrinkles   b) cleanse the skin
    c) strengthen facial   d) reduce fat cells
        muscles   _____

62. Preparations that temporarily remove superfluous hair
    by dissolving it at the skin line are:
    a) depilatories   b) epilators
    c) razors   d) waxes   _____

63. Scalp lotions and ointments usually contain:
    a) surfactants   b) witch hazel
    c) alcohol   d) medicinal agents   _____

64. The primary ingredient in styptic powder or liquid is:
    a) talc   b) alum
    c) alcohol   d) witch hazel   _____

65. Witch hazel is a solution that acts as a/an:
    a) astringent   b) emulsion
    c) suspension   d) acid   _____

66. All electrical appliances used in the barbershop should be:
    a) Barber Board certified   b) FDA certified
    c) UL certified   d) OSHA certified   _____

67. Electric clippers and hair dryers are examples of
    barbering tools that use:
    a) alternating current   b) converted current
    c) direct current   d) rectified current   _____

68. The different types of currents used in facial and scalp
    treatments are called:
    a) units   b) AC
    c) modalities   d) DC   _____

69. An applicator that directs electric current from the
    machine to the client's skin is a/an:
    a) conductor   b) modality
    c) electrode   d) massager   _____

70. The high-frequency current commonly used in the
    barbershop is the:
    a) d'Arsonval current   b) Oudin current
    c) sinusoidal current   d) tesla current   _____

71. For a stimulating effect, the high-frequency electrode is:
    a) slightly lifted from   b) in close contact with
        the skin   the skin
    c) held by the client   d) turned very low   _____

72. Ultraviolet rays produce:
    a) heat
    b) germicidal reactions
    c) chemical reactions
    d) b and c
    _____

73. Ultraviolet rays are also known as:
    a) actinic rays
    b) cold rays
    c) tanning rays
    d) a, b, and c
    _____

74. The outer protective layer of the skin is called the scarf skin or the:
    a) dermis
    b) adipose tissue
    c) epidermis
    d) subcutaneous tissue
    _____

75. The growth of the epidermis starts in the:
    a) stratum lucidum
    b) stratum germinativum
    c) stratum corneum
    d) stratum granulosum
    _____

76. The color of the skin is due to the amount of blood it contains and:
    a) keratin
    b) moisture
    c) fat
    d) melanin
    _____

77. The epidermis contains:
    a) blood vessels
    b) small nerve endings
    c) adipose tissue
    d) subcutaneous tissue
    _____

78. The dermis is also known as the corium, cutis, derma, and:
    a) cuticle
    b) false skin
    c) true skin
    d) fatty tissue
    _____

79. Subcutaneous tissue is also known as:
    a) muscle tissue
    b) soft tissue
    c) adipose tissue
    d) hard tissue
    _____

80. The sebaceous glands are duct glands that secrete:
    a) melanin
    b) sebum
    c) saliva
    d) perspiration
    _____

81. The duct of an oil gland empties into the:
    a) blood vessel
    b) hair follicle
    c) sweat pore
    d) hair papilla
    _____

82. Examples of primary skin lesions include the following *except:*
    a) bulla, cyst, macule
    b) vesicle, wheal
    c) papule, pustule, tubercle
    d) scar, fissure, keloid
    _____

83. Examples of secondary lesions include the following *except:*
    a) bulla, cyst, macule   b) scale, scab
    c) excoriation, crust   d) scar, fissure, keloid   _____

84. A skin wart is known as a:
    a) keloid   b) keratoma
    c) verruca   d) nevus   _____

85. The general term for an inflammatory condition of the skin is:
    a) trichology   b) dermatology
    c) histology   d) dermatitis   _____

86. Milia is the technical name for a:
    a) whitehead   b) pimple
    c) blackhead   d) dry skin   _____

87. Acne is a disorder of the:
    a) sweat glands   b) oil glands
    c) intestinal glands   d) stomach glands   _____

88. An inflammatory skin disease that may be acute or chronic with dry or moist lesions is:
    a) eczema   b) seborrhea
    c) psoriasis   d) herpes simplex   _____

89. A recurring viral infection that produces fever blisters or cold sores is:
    a) eczema   b) herpes simplex
    c) psoriasis   d) dermatitis venenata   _____

90. The most common and least severe type of skin cancer is:
    a) squamous cell   b) malignant melanoma
    carcinoma
    c) basal cell carcinoma   d) melanoma   _____

91. Hair is chiefly composed of a horny substance called:
    a) hemoglobin   b) melanin
    c) keratin   d) calcium   _____

92. That portion of the hair that extends beyond the skin surface is called the:
    a) hair root   b) hair bulb
    c) hair shaft   d) hair papilla   _____

93. A small, cone-shaped elevation at the base of the hair follicle is called the:
    a) dermal papilla
    b) hair bulb
    c) hair shaft
    d) hair follicle ____

94. Glands that excrete perspiration through the skin pores are called:
    a) sudoriferous glands
    b) follicle glands
    c) sebaceous glands
    d) excretion glands ____

95. The three main layers of the hair shaft are the:
    a) cuticle, cortex, and medulla
    b) follicle, root, and bulb
    c) root, bulb, and dermal papilla
    d) follicle, root, and papilla ____

96. That portion of the hair that provides strength, elasticity, and natural color is the:
    a) medulla
    b) hair shaft
    c) cortex
    d) cuticle ____

97. Hair cells mature in the follicle through a process known as:
    a) cauterization
    b) dissemination
    c) keratinization
    d) propagation ____

98. Hair grows an average of:
    a) $\frac{1}{4}$ inch per month
    b) $\frac{1}{2}$ inch per month
    c) $\frac{3}{4}$ inch per month
    d) 1 inch per month ____

99. The term used to indicate the number of individual hair strands per square inch of scalp area is:
    a) density
    b) porosity
    c) elasticity
    d) texture ____

100. The ability of the hair to absorb moisture determines its:
    a) level of density
    b) level of porosity
    c) level of elasticity
    d) variation in texture ____

101. Alopecia is the technical term for any abnormal type of:
    a) hair loss
    b) skin inflammation
    c) oil gland disorder
    d) sweat gland disorder ____

102. Common scalp disorders include dandruff, vegetable and animal parasitic infections, and:
    a) diplococcal infections
    b) streptococcal infections
    c) staphylococcal infections
    d) pediculosis infestations ____

172

103. Small, white scales appearing on the scalp and hair is a sign of:
    a) dermatitis   b) eczema
    c) herpes simplex   d) pityriasis   _____

104. Ringworm of the scalp is the common name for:
    a) tinea   b) tinea favosa
    c) tinea capitis   d) tinea sycosis   _____

105. All forms of tinea are:
    a) nontreatable   b) contagious
    c) noncontagious   d) treatable by the barber   _____

106. Pediculosis and scabies are:
    a) nontreatable   b) not contagious
    c) contagious   d) treatable by the barber   _____
        infestations

107. Inflammations of the follicle caused by bacteria or irritation may be signs of:
    a) folliculitis   b) pseudofolliculitis barbae
    c) a or b   d) neither a nor b   _____

108. The main purpose of a shampoo is to:
    a) make hair easier   b) cleanse the hair and
        to comb   scalp
    c) treat alopecia areata   d) soften the scalp   _____

109. Solutions that harden, shrink, or constrict the cuticle scales usually have a/an:
    a) acidic pH level   b) neutral pH level
    c) alkaline pH level   d) harsh pH level   _____

110. The portion of the shampoo molecule that attracts dirt and repels water is the:
    a) head   b) middle
    c) belly   d) tail   _____

111. Hair loss characterized by the sudden falling out of hair in round patches is called:
    a) androgenic alopecia   b) alopecia senilis
    c) alopecia areata   d) alopecia syphilitica   _____

112. Rinses that are formulated to control minor dandruff and scalp conditions are:
    a) water rinses   b) bluing rinses
    c) medicated rinses   d) tonic rinses   _____

113. A cosmetic solution that can stimulate the scalp, correct a scalp condition, or be used as a grooming aid is a:
    a) hair tonic
    b) styling spray
    c) conditioner
    d) scalp ointment _____

114. The purpose of a towel or neck strip between the drape and the client's skin is to:
    a) maintain sanitation standards
    b) conform to state barber laws
    c) prevent drape contact with client's skin
    d) a, b, and c _____

115. The two methods employed by barbers to perform a shampoo service are the:
    a) upright and reclined methods
    b) inclined and reclined methods
    c) tub and shower methods
    d) backward and reclined methods _____

116. Shampoo and scalp manipulations are performed with:
    a) the cushions of the fingertips
    b) fingernails
    c) rubber gloves
    d) disposable gloves _____

117. Scalp massage should be performed with:
    a) fast motion and no pressure
    b) slow motion and no pressure
    c) continuous, even motion and pressure
    d) fast motion and heavy pressure _____

118. Barbers are qualified to perform treatments for the following *except:*
    a) dry scalp
    b) oily scalp and hair
    c) dandruff
    d) parasitic or staphylococcus conditions _____

119. Cleansing the hair without soap and water can be accomplished by using a/an:
    a) liquid dry shampoo
    b) powder dry shampoo
    c) evaporating shampoo
    d) a or b _____

120. Conditions that may prohibit a facial massage include the following *except:*
    a) normal blood pressure
    b) severe skin lesions
    c) skin inflammation
    d) high blood pressure _____

121. A point on the skin where pressure or stimulation will cause contraction of the muscle is a:
    a) motor point
    b) trigger point
    c) sensory point
    d) secretory point
    _____

122. Effleurage is used in massage for its:
    a) stimulating effects
    b) soothing and relaxing effects
    c) heating effects
    d) frictional effects
    _____

123. Facials performed in the barbershop are considered to be either:
    a) preventive or corrective
    b) corrective or medicinal
    c) preventive or medicinal
    d) corrective or therapeutic
    _____

124. The four skin types include dry, normal, combination, and:
    a) sensitive
    b) allergic
    c) irritated
    d) oily
    _____

125. A scalp steam *is not* used to:
    a) relax and open the pores
    b) close the pores
    c) soften the scalp
    d) increase blood circulation
    _____

126. All of the following may cause ingrown hairs *except:*
    a) excessively close shaving
    b) shear cutting
    c) excessive pressure
    d) improper use of tweezers, razor, or trimmers
    _____

127. To achieve the best cutting stroke, the razor must glide over the surface at an angle:
    a) with the grain of the hair
    b) against the grain of the hair
    c) across the grain of the hair
    d) diagonal to the grain of the hair
    _____

128. When shaving, a gliding stroke directed away from the barber is used with the:
    a) freehand stroke
    b) backhand stroke
    c) cutting stroke
    d) reverse freehand stroke
    _____

129. The once-over shave requires several strokes with each shaving movement:
    a) against the grain of the hair
    b) with the grain of the hair
    c) across the grain of the hair
    d) diagonal to the grain of the hair
    _____

130. Ingrown hairs are a common problem of:
    a) straight hair   b) wavy hair
    c) coarse hair   d) curly hair   _____

131. A tapered haircut is longer in the crown and top areas and:
    a) shorter at the nape   b) uniform at the nape
    c) longer at the nape   d) neither a, b, or c   _____

132. The removal of excess bulk from the hair is called:
    a) slithering   b) dethickening
    c) customizing   d) thinning   _____

133. When using the shear-over-comb technique, the hair is placed in position for cutting by:
    a) combing through it   b) holding hair between
                                 the fingers
    c) brushing through   d) rolling the
       the hair   comb out   _____

134. The standard clipper cutting techniques are the:
    a) freehand and   b) clipper-over-comb
       backhand   and freehand
    c) freehand and   d) clipper-over-comb
       underhand   and backhand   _____

135. The type of cutting method that can help make resistant hair textures more manageable is:
    a) razor cutting   b) clipper cutting
    c) shear cutting   d) hair singeing   _____

136. Razor cutting requires that the hair be:
    a) chemically processed   b) clean and damp
    c) clean and dry   d) misted   _____

137. Shaving the sides of the neck and across the nape with a razor is called a/an:
    a) extra service   b) outline shave
    c) neck shave   d) hairline shave   _____

138. Hair replacement techniques include toupees or hairpieces and the following *except:*
    a) certain drugs   b) chemical processes
    c) surgical hair   d) scalp reduction
       transplantation   _____

139. Hairpieces made of human hair must be:
   a) shampooed and conditioned
   b) dry cleaned
   c) washed with warm water
   d) cleaned with acetone
   _____

138. Hairpieces may be cut and blended with shears or a/an:
   a) clipper
   b) outliner
   c) razor
   d) edger
   _____

141. The process used to chemically restructure straight hair into a wave pattern is:
   a) permanent waving
   b) haircoloring
   c) reformation curls
   d) hair relaxing
   _____

142. A reformation curl is also known as the following except:
   a) chemical blow-out
   b) Jheri curl
   c) soft-curl perm
   d) a curl
   _____

143. The process used to rearrange overcurly hair into a straightened hair form is known as:
   a) permanent wave
   b) a curl
   c) reformation curl
   d) chemical hair relaxing
   _____

144. The two layers of the hair most affected by chemical texture services are the:
   a) cortex and medulla
   b) cortex and cuticle
   c) medulla and cuticle
   d) cortex and hair root
   _____

145. The partial or total removal of natural pigment or artificial color from the hair is called:
   a) hair lightening
   b) hair stripping
   c) haircoloring
   d) hair dying
   _____

146. The four classifications of haircoloring products include temporary and the following except:
   a) semipermanent
   b) permanent
   c) demipermanent
   d) temporary semipermanent
   _____

147. Temporary haircolor products are a type of:
   a) oxidation color
   b) penetrating color
   c) nonoxidation color
   d) self-penetrating color
   _____

148. Characteristics of permanent haircolor products include the following except:
   a) mixed with hydrogen peroxide
   b) do not need retouch applications
   c) deposit and lift
   d) are penetrating tints
   _____

149. The technical term applied to any deformity or disease of the nail is:
    a) onychosis
    b) melanonychia
    c) eponychium
    d) leukonychia
    _____

150. Business operating expenses are also known as:
    a) overhead
    b) accounts receivables
    c) credits
    d) tax rebates
    _____

SAMPLE STATE BOARD EXAMINATION TEST 3

1. The first state to pass a barber license law was:
   - a) Minnesota
   - b) New York
   - c) Illinois
   - d) Ohio _____

2. Barber-surgeons participated in the practice of:
   - a) bloodletting
   - b) teeth pulling
   - c) surgery
   - d) a, b, and c _____

3. State barber boards are primarily interested in maintaining high standards of:
   - a) appliances
   - b) tools
   - c) products
   - d) competency _____

4. One key function of state barber boards is to protect the health, safety, and welfare of the:
   - a) profession
   - b) barbers
   - c) public
   - d) board members _____

5. Proper behavior and business dealings with employers, clients, and coworkers is called:
   - a) professional technique
   - b) professional ethics
   - c) career guidance
   - d) behavioral characteristics _____

6. Pathogenic bacteria produce:
   - a) health
   - b) disease
   - c) antitoxins
   - d) beneficial effects _____

7. Pus-forming organisms that grow in clusters and cause abscesses, pustules, pimples, and boils are:
   - a) staphylococci bacteria
   - b) streptococci bacteria
   - c) diplococci bacteria
   - d) spirilla bacteria _____

8. Pustules and boils contain:
   - a) nonpathogenic organisms
   - b) pathogenic bacteria
   - c) sweat
   - d) ringworm _____

9. The presence of pus is a sign of:
   - a) infection
   - b) impurities
   - c) immunity
   - d) healing _____

10. Ringworm is caused by a/an:
    - a) animal parasite
    - b) poison ivy
    - c) bacterial parasite
    - d) plant parasite _____

11. Pediculosis is caused by:
    a) the itch mite
    b) the body or head louse
    c) scabies
    d) ringworm
    _____

12. The virus that causes AIDS is:
    a) HIV
    b) HIB
    c) ARC
    d) STD
    _____

13. The most likely manner in which HIV may be transmitted in the barbershop is by:
    a) shaking hands with an infected person
    b) blood to blood contact with an infected person
    c) using a soiled headrest
    d) using a sanitized comb
    _____

14. The removal of pathogens from tools and surfaces is known as:
    a) decontamination
    b) contamination
    c) sepsis
    d) cleaning
    _____

15. The process of thoroughly cleaning a tool or surface to its optimum level of decontamination in the barbershop is known as:
    a) sterilization
    b) sanitizer
    c) disinfectant
    d) disinfection or sanitation
    _____

16. State barber boards and health departments require only:
    a) sterilization procedures
    b) sanitation procedures
    c) disinfection procedures
    d) disinfection and sanitation procedures
    _____

17. A disinfectant that contains the properties of a bactericide, fungicide, pseudomonacide, virucide, and tuberculocide is considered to be a/an:
    a) minimal disinfectant
    b) hospital level disinfectant
    c) deodorizer
    d) antiseptic
    _____

18. Antiseptics may be used on:
    a) the skin
    b) cutting implements
    c) dirty floors
    d) brushes and combs
    _____

19. For effective sanitization, the minimum strength of a quat solution used to sanitize implements is:
    a) 10%
    b) 1:2000
    c) 1:1000
    d) 20%
    _____

20. A wet sanitizer should contain:
    - a) a disinfectant solution
    - b) 30% alcohol
    - c) an antiseptic solution
    - d) 2% formalin   _____

21. The Occupational Safety and Health Administration (OSHA) regulates and enforces safety and health in the workplace by:
    - a) setting safety standards
    - b) selling safe products
    - c) causing worker injury
    - d) importing products   _____

22. Keep clean towels:
    - a) near dirty towels
    - b) in a clean, open cabinet
    - c) in a clean, closed cabinet
    - d) on a nearby shelf   _____

23. Barbers should wash their hands:
    - a) in the morning
    - b) when they get dirty
    - c) morning and afternoon
    - d) before and after serving each client   _____

24. Implements must be cleaned prior to immersion in a disinfectant solution to:
    - a) avoid solution contamination
    - b) comply with state board rules
    - c) comply with sanitation procedures
    - d) a, b, and c   _____

25. When a blood spill occurs, employ:
    - a) a doctor
    - b) safety precautions
    - c) universal precautions
    - d) decontamination   _____

26. Cream should be removed from jars with:
    - a) the end of a used towel
    - b) tips of fingers
    - c) a clean spatula
    - d) a comedone extractor   _____

27. Hair or other waste materials on the floor of a barbershop should be:
    - a) swept into a corner
    - b) placed in a closed container
    - c) placed in a garbage can
    - d) swept up at the end of the day   _____

28. Small nicks or cuts should be cleansed and treated with:
    - a) a band aid
    - b) soap and water
    - c) styptic powder
    - d) styptic pencil   _____

29. The most desirable type of hair comb is made of:
    a) plastic
    b) metal
    c) bone
    d) hard rubber
    _____

30. The French type of haircutting shears:
    a) has no finger brace
    b) has one finger brace
    c) has two finger braces
    d) does not have a shank
    _____

31. When holding haircutting shears properly, the barber places the thumb in the thumb grip of the:
    a) shank
    b) still blade
    c) moving blade
    d) finger grip
    _____

32. Electric clippers are driven by rotary motor, magnetic motor, or:
    a) circular motor
    b) pivot motor
    c) vibratory motor
    d) motor action
    _____

33. Headrest covers must be changed:
    a) for each client
    b) whenever they get soiled
    c) for every three clients
    d) for every other client
    _____

34. The clipper blade size that leaves the hair the longest is:
    a) size 1
    b) size 2
    c) size $1\frac{1}{2}$
    d) size 3
    _____

35. The first step in sanitizing clippers and trimmers is to:
    a) brush off hair particles
    b) immerse blades in blade wash
    c) immerse blades in water
    d) spray with disinfectant
    _____

36. The grind of a razor refers to the shape of the:
    a) tang
    b) heel
    c) blade
    d) handle
    _____

37. The size of a razor refers is measured by the blade's:
    a) length
    b) thickness
    c) sharpness
    d) length and width
    _____

38. A crocus finish on the blade of a razor is also known as:
    a) nickel-plated finish
    b) silver-plated finish
    c) plain steel finish
    d) polished steel finish
    _____

39. The purpose of a hone is to:
    a) grind the razor's edge
    b) smooth the razor's edge
    c) polish the razor's edge
    d) align the razor's cutting teeth
    _____

40. The purpose of a strop is to:
    a) grind the razor's edge
    b) smooth the razor's edge
    c) polish the razor's edge
    d) impart a cutting edge to the razor

    _____

41. The shell or Russian shell strop is created from:
    a) the rump area of the horse
    b) cowhide
    c) synthetic materials
    d) canvas

    _____

42. The direction used in razor stropping is:
    a) the same as that used in honing
    b) in a counter-clockwise direction
    c) the reverse of that used in honing
    d) in a clockwise direction

    _____

43. Clipper blades are usually made of:
    a) tempered nickel
    b) chrome
    c) hard rubber
    d) carbon steel

    _____

44. The least acceptable method of removing loose hair after a haircut is the:
    a) small electric vacuum
    b) clean towel, properly folded
    c) unsanitized neck duster
    d) paper neck strips

    _____

45. The skull consists of eight cranial bones and:
    a) 8 facial bones
    b) 10 facial bones
    c) 12 facial bones
    d) 14 facial bones

    _____

46. The occipital bone forms the back and base of the:
    a) neck
    b) cranium
    c) upper jaw
    d) forehead

    _____

47. The least fixed attachment of a muscle to the bone is called the:
    a) origin
    b) insertion
    c) joint
    d) ligament

    _____

48. Muscle tissue may be stimulated by massage, electric current, and:
    a) heat and light rays
    b) nerve impulses and chemicals
    c) moist heat
    d) a, b, and c

    _____

49. The parietal bones form the top and sides of the:
    a) face
    b) cranium
    c) cheeks
    d) neck

    _____

50. Nerves may be stimulated by high-frequency current, moist heat, and:
    a) chemicals
    b) light and heat rays
    c) massage
    d) a, b , and c   _____

51. The main sources of blood to the head, face, and neck are supplied by the
    a) jugular veins
    b) common carotid arteries
    c) arteries
    d) veins   _____

52. The skin and its appendages make up the:
    a) integumentary system
    b) endocrine system
    c) circulatory system
    d) capillary system   _____

53. Twelve pairs of cranial nerves branch out from the brain and reach parts of the:
    a) arms and hands
    b) legs and feet
    c) abdomen and back
    d) head, face, and neck   _____

54. The liquid that is considered to be a universal solvent is:
    a) alcohol
    b) peroxide
    c) bleach
    d) water   _____

55. The best type of water to use in the barbershop is:
    a) distilled water
    b) mineral water
    c) soft water
    d) hard water   _____

56. The pH of a solution measures its degree of:
    a) softness or hardness
    b) acidity or alkalinity
    c) heat or cold level
    d) neutrality   _____

57. The pH range of hair and skin is:
    a) 3.5 to 4.5
    b) 4.5 to 6.5
    c) 4.5 to 5.5
    d) 5.5 to 6.5   _____

58. An example of a suspension is:
    a) a quat solution
    b) hair oil tonic
    c) witch hazel
    d) shampoo   _____

59. A mixture of two or more substances that is made by dissolving a solid, liquid, or gaseous substance in another substance is known as a/an:
    a) solution
    b) ointment
    c) suspension
    d) powder   _____

60. Cosmetic preparations that will cause the contraction of skin tissues are:
    a) fresheners
    b) astringents
    c) facial toners
    d) a, b, and c   _____

61. The basic purpose of a cold cream is to:
    a) eradicate wrinkles
    b) cleanse the skin
    c) strengthen facial muscles
    d) reduce fat cells
    _____

62. Preparations that temporarily remove superfluous hair by dissolving it at the skin line are:
    a) depilatories
    b) epilators
    c) razors
    d) waxes
    _____

63. Scalp lotions and ointments usually contain:
    a) surfactants
    b) witch hazel
    c) alcohol
    d) medicinal agents
    _____

64. The primary ingredient in styptic powder or liquid is:
    a) talc
    b) alum
    c) alcohol
    d) witch hazel
    _____

65. Witch hazel is a solution that acts as a/an:
    a) astringent
    b) emulsion
    c) suspension
    d) acid
    _____

66. All electrical appliances used in the barbershop should be:
    a) Barber Board certified
    b) FDA certified
    c) UL certified
    d) OSHA certified
    _____

67. Electric clippers and hair dryers are examples of barbering tools that use:
    a) alternating current
    b) converted current
    c) direct current
    d) rectified current
    _____

68. The different types of currents used in facial and scalp treatments are called:
    a) units
    b) AC
    c) modalities
    d) DC
    _____

69. An applicator that directs electric current from the machine to the client's skin is a/an:
    a) conductor
    b) modality
    c) electrode
    d) massager
    _____

70. The high-frequency current commonly used in the barbershop is the:
    a) d'Arsonval current
    b) Oudin current
    c) sinusoidal current
    d) tesla current
    _____

71. For a stimulating effect, the high-frequency electrode is:
    a) slightly lifted from the skin
    b) in close contact with the skin
    c) held by the client
    d) turned very low
    _____

72. Ultraviolet rays produce:
    a) heat
    b) germicidal reactions
    c) chemical reactions
    d) b and c
    _____

73. Ultraviolet rays are also known as:
    a) actinic rays
    b) cold rays
    c) tanning rays
    d) a, b, and c
    _____

74. The outer protective layer of the skin is called the scarf skin or the:
    a) dermis
    b) adipose tissue
    c) epidermis
    d) subcutaneous tissue
    _____

75. The layer of the epidermis that is continually shed is the:
    a) stratum lucidum
    b) stratum germinativum
    c) stratum corneum
    d) stratum granulosum
    _____

76. The color of the skin is due to the amount of blood it contains and:
    a) keratin
    b) moisture
    c) fat
    d) melanin
    _____

77. The epidermis contains:
    a) blood vessels
    b) small nerve endings
    c) adipose tissue
    d) subcutaneous tissue
    _____

78. The dermis is also known as the corium, cutis, derma, and:
    a) cuticle
    b) false skin
    c) true skin
    d) fatty tissue
    _____

79. Subcutaneous tissue is also known as:
    a) muscle tissue
    b) soft tissue
    c) adipose tissue
    d) hard tissue
    _____

80. The sebaceous glands are duct glands that secrete:
    a) melanin
    b) sebum
    c) saliva
    d) perspiration
    _____

81. The duct of an oil gland empties into the:
    a) blood vessel
    b) hair follicle
    c) sweat pore
    d) hair papilla
    _____

82. Examples of primary skin lesions include the following *except:*
    a) bulla, cyst, macule
    b) vesicle, wheal
    c) papule, pustule, tubercle
    d) scar, fissure, keloid
    _____

83. Examples of secondary lesions include the following *except:*
    a) bulla, cyst, macule   b) scale, scab
    c) excoriation, crust   d) scar, fissure, keloid   _____

84. A skin wart is known as a:
    a) keloid   b) keratoma
    c) verruca   d) nevus   _____

85. The general term for an inflammatory condition of the skin is:
    a) trichology   b) dermatology
    c) histology   d) dermatitis   _____

86. Milia is the technical name for a:
    a) whitehead   b) pimple
    c) blackhead   d) dry skin   _____

87. Acne is a disorder of the:
    a) sweat glands   b) oil glands
    c) intestinal glands   d) stomach glands   _____

88. A chronic, inflammatory skin disease with dry red patches and coarse silvery scales is:
    a) eczema   b) herpes simplex
    c) psoriasis   d) dermatitis venenata   _____

89. A recurring viral infection that produces fever blisters or cold sores is:
    a) eczema   b) herpes simplex
    c) psoriasis   d) dermatitis venenata   _____

90. The most common and least severe type of skin cancer is:
    a) squamous cell carcinoma   b) malignant melanoma
    c) basal cell carcinoma   d) melanoma   _____

91. Hair is chiefly composed of a horny substance called:
    a) hemoglobin   b) melanin
    c) keratin   d) calcium   _____

92. That portion of the hair that extends beyond the skin surface is called the:
    a) hair root   b) hair bulb
    c) hair shaft   d) hair papilla   _____

93. A small, cone-shaped elevation at the base of the hair follicle is called the:
    a) dermal papilla   b) hair bulb
    c) hair shaft   d) hair follicle   _____

94. Glands that excrete perspiration through the skin pores are called:
    a) sudoriferous glands
    b) follicle glands
    c) sebaceous glands
    d) excretion glands
    _____

95. The three main layers of the hair shaft are the:
    a) cuticle, cortex, and medulla
    b) follicle, root, and bulb
    c) root, bulb, and dermal papilla
    d) follicle, root, and papilla
    _____

96. That portion of the hair that provides strength, elasticity, and natural color is the:
    a) medulla
    b) hair shaft
    c) cortex
    d) cuticle
    _____

97. Hair cells mature in the follicle through a process known as:
    a) cauterization
    b) dissemination
    c) keratinization
    d) propagation
    _____

98. Hair grows an average of:
    a) $\frac{1}{4}$ inch per month
    b) $\frac{1}{2}$ inch per month
    c) $\frac{3}{4}$ inch per month
    d) 1 inch per month
    _____

99. The term used to indicate the number of individual hair strands per square inch of scalp area is:
    a) density
    b) porosity
    c) elasticity
    d) texture
    _____

100. The ability of the hair to absorb moisture determines its:
    a) level of density
    b) level of porosity
    c) level of elasticity
    d) variation in texture
    _____

101. Alopecia is the technical term for any abnormal type of:
    a) hair loss
    b) skin inflammation
    c) oil gland disorder
    d) sweat gland disorder
    _____

102. Common scalp disorders include dandruff, vegetable and animal parasitic infections, and:
    a) diplococcal infections
    b) streptococcal infections
    c) staphylococcal infections
    d) pediculosis infestations
    _____

103. Small, white scales appearing on the scalp and hair is a sign of:
    a) dermatitis
    b) eczema
    c) herpes simplex
    d) pityriasis
    _____

104. Ringworm of the scalp is the common name for:
    a) tinea
    b) tinea favosa
    c) tinea capitis
    d) tinea sycosis
    _____

105. All forms of tinea are:
    a) nontreatable
    b) contagious
    c) noncontagious
    d) treatable by the barber
    _____

106. Pediculosis and scabies are:
    a) nontreatable
    b) not contagious
    c) contagious
       infestations
    d) treatable by the barber
    _____

107. Inflammations of the follicle caused by bacteria or
    irritation may be signs of:
    a) folliculitis
    b) pseudofolliculitis barbae
    c) a or b
    d) neither a nor b
    _____

108. The main purpose of a shampoo is to:
    a) make hair easier
       to comb
    b) cleanse the hair
       and scalp
    c) treat alopecia areata
    d) soften the scalp
    _____

109. Solutions that harden, shrink, or constrict the cuticle
    scales usually have a/an:
    a) acidic pH level
    b) neutral pH level
    c) alkaline pH level
    d) harsh pH level
    _____

110. The portion of the shampoo molecule that attracts dirt
    and repels water is the:
    a) head
    b) middle
    c) belly
    d) tail
    _____

111. Hair loss characterized by the sudden falling out of hair
    in round patches is called:
    a) androgenic alopecia
    b) alopecia senilis
    c) alopecia areata
    d) alopecia syphilitica
    _____

112. Rinses that are formulated to control minor dandruff
    and scalp conditions are:
    a) water rinses
    b) bluing rinses
    c) medicated rinses
    d) tonic rinses
    _____

113. A cosmetic solution that can stimulate the scalp,
    correct a scalp condition, or be used as a grooming
    aid is a:
    a) hair tonic
    b) styling spray
    c) conditioner
    d) scalp ointment
    _____

114. The purpose of a towel or neck strip between the drape and the client's skin is to:
    a) maintain sanitation standards
    b) conform to state barber laws
    c) prevent drape contact with client's skin
    d) a, b, and c
    _____

115. The two methods employed by barbers to perform a shampoo service are the:
    a) upright and reclined methods
    b) inclined and reclined methods
    c) tub and shower methods
    d) backward and reclined methods
    _____

116. Shampoo and scalp manipulations are performed with:
    a) the cushions of the fingertips
    b) fingernails
    c) rubber gloves
    d) disposable gloves
    _____

117. Scalp massage should be performed with:
    a) fast motion and no pressure
    b) slow motion and no pressure
    c) continuous, even motion and pressure
    d) fast motion and heavy pressure
    _____

118. Barbers are qualified to perform treatments for the following *except:*
    a) dry scalp
    b) oily scalp and hair
    c) dandruff
    d) parasitic or staphylococcus conditions
    _____

119. Cleansing the hair without soap and water can be accomplished by using a/an:
    a) liquid dry shampoo
    b) powder dry shampoo
    c) evaporating shampoo
    d) a or b
    _____

120. Conditions that may prohibit a facial massage include the following *except:*
    a) normal blood pressure
    b) severe skin lesions
    c) skin inflammation
    d) high blood pressure
    _____

121. A point on the skin where pressure or stimulation will cause contraction of the muscle is a/an:
    a) motor point
    b) trigger point
    c) sensory point
    d) secretory point
    _____

122. Pétrissage is the type of massage movement involving:
    a) friction
    b) percussion
    c) kneading or pinching
    d) tapotement
    _____

123. Effleurage is used in massage for its:
    a) stimulating effects   b) soothing and relaxing
                                    effects
    c) heating effects   d) frictional effects   _____

124. The four skin types include dry, normal, oily, and:
    a) sensitive   b) allergic
    c) irritated   d) combination   _____

125. A scalp steam *is not* used to:
    a) relax and open   b) close the pores
       the pores
    c) soften the scalp   d) increase blood circulation   _____

126. All of the following may cause ingrown hairs *except:*
    a) excessively close   b) shear cutting
       shaving
    c) excessive pressure   d) improper use of tweezers,
                                      razor, or trimmers   _____

127. To achieve the best cutting stroke, the razor must glide
over the surface at an angle:
    a) with the grain   b) against the grain
       of the hair   of the hair
    c) across the grain   d) diagonal to the grain
       of the hair   of the hair   _____

128. When shaving, a gliding stroke directed away from the
barber is used with the:
    a) freehand stroke   b) backhand stroke
    c) cutting stroke   d) reverse freehand stroke   _____

129. The once-over shave requires several strokes with each
shaving movement:
    a) against the grain   b) with the grain
       of the hair   of the hair
    c) across the grain   d) diagonal to the grain
       of the hair   of the hair   _____

130. Ingrown hairs are a common problem of:
    a) straight hair   b) wavy hair
    c) coarse hair   d) curly hair   _____

131. A tapered haircut is longer in the crown and top areas
and:
    a) shorter at the nape   b) uniform at the nape
    c) longer at the nape   d) neither a, b, or c   _____

132. The removal of excess bulk from the hair is called:
    a) slithering
    b) dethickening
    c) customizing
    d) thinning
    _____

133. When using the shear-over-comb technique, the hair is placed in position for cutting by:
    a) combing through it
    b) holding it between the fingers
    c) brushing through the hair
    d) rolling the comb out
    _____

134. The standard clipper cutting techniques are the:
    a) freehand and backhand
    b) clipper-over-comb and freehand
    c) freehand and underhand
    d) clipper-over-comb and backhand
    _____

135. The type of cutting method that can help make resistant hair textures more manageable is:
    a) razor cutting
    b) clipper cutting
    c) shear cutting
    d) hair singeing
    _____

136. Razor cutting requires that the hair be:
    a) chemically processed
    b) clean and damp
    c) clean and dry
    d) misted
    _____

137. Shaving the sides of the neck and across the nape with a razor is called a/an:
    a) extra service
    b) outline shave
    c) neck shave
    d) hairline shave
    _____

138. Hair replacement techniques include toupees or hairpieces and the following *except:*
    a) certain drugs
    b) chemical processes
    c) surgical hair transplantation
    d) scalp reduction
    _____

139. Hairpieces made of human hair must be:
    a) shampooed and conditioned
    b) dry cleaned
    c) washed with warm water
    d) cleaned with acetone
    _____

140. Hairpieces may be cut and blended with shears or a/an:
    a) clipper
    b) outliner
    c) razor
    d) edger
    _____

141. The process used to chemically restructure straight hair into a wave pattern is:
   a) permanent waving b) haircoloring
   c) reformation curls d) hair relaxing _____

142. A soft-curl perm is also known as the following *except:*
   a) chemical blow-out b) Jheri curl
   c) reformation curl d) a curl _____

143. The process used to rearrange over-curly hair into a straightened hair form is known as:
   a) permanent wave b) a curl
   c) reformation curl d) chemical hair relaxing _____

144. The two layers of the hair most affected by chemical texture services are the:
   a) cortex and medulla b) cortex and cuticle
   c) medulla and cuticle d) cortex and hair root _____

145. The partial or total removal of natural pigment or artificial color from the hair is called:
   a) hair lightening b) hair stripping
   c) haircoloring d) hair dying _____

146. The four classifications of haircoloring products include temporary and the following *except:*
   a) semipermanent b) permanent
   c) demipermanent d) temporary semipermanent _____

147. Temporary haircolor products are a type of:
   a) oxidation color b) penetrating color
   c) nonoxidation color d) self-penetrating color _____

148. Characteristics of permanent haircolor products include the following *except:*
   a) mixed with hydrogen peroxide b) do not need retouch applications
   c) deposit and lift d) are penetrating tints _____

149. The technical term applied to any deformity or disease of the nail is:
   a) onychosis b) melanonychia
   c) eponychium d) leukonychia _____

150. Business operating expenses are also known as:
   a) overhead b) accounts receivables
   c) credits d) tax rebates _____

Answers to Chapter Review Tests

CHAPTER 1: STUDY SKILLS

1. c	2. d	3. c	4. b
5. c	6. b	7. a	8. d

CHAPTER 2: THE HISTORY OF BARBERING

1. b	2. d	3. c	4. b	5. c
6. d	7. a	8. b	9. b	10. c
11. a	12. d	13. b	14. c	15. b
16. b	17. c	18. c	19. c	20. a
21. a	22. b	23. c	24. d	25. c

CHAPTER 3: YOUR PROFESSIONAL IMAGE

1. c	2. b	3. a	4. b	5. d
6. c	7. a	8. c	9. b	10. d
11. a	12. c	13. c	14. c	15. a
16. d	17. d	18. b	19. a	20. a
21. c	22. b	23. b	24. d	25. c
26. b	27. c	28. d	29. b	30. d
31. a	32. d	33. b	34. c	35. a
36. c	37. c	38. a	39. d	40. d
41. a	42. d	43. a	44. c	45. d
46. b	47. a	48. c	49. d	50. d

CHAPTER 4: BACTERIOLOGY

1. c	2. a	3. c	4. b	5. b
6. c	7. c	8. a	9. a	10. c
11. b	12. b	13. a	14. c	15. b
16. d	17. b	18. c	19. b	20. a
21. c	22. b	23. a	24. c	25. b
26. a	27. b	28. b	29. c	30. d
31. b	32. c	33. b	34. a	35. c
36. c	37. b	38. d	39. b	40. a
41. d	42. b	43. d	44. c	45. b
46. c	47. d	48. b	49. c	50. a

CHAPTER 5: INFECTION CONTROL & SAFE WORK PRACTICES

1. c	2. a	3. d	4. d	5. a
6. d	7. d	8. b	9. c	10. b
11. a	12. c	13. c	14. c	15. c
16. a	17. c	18. c	19. d	20. a
21. b	22. c	23. c	24. a	25. b
26. b	27. d	28. a	29. b	30. d
31. c	32. c	33. b	34. c	35. c
36. d	37. a	38. c	39. c	40. d
41. c	42. c	43. c	44. c	45. d
46. d	47. b	48. c	49. c	50. b
51. a	52. c	53. c	54. c	55. b
56. b	57. a	58. a	59. c	60. c

CHAPTER 6: IMPLEMENTS, TOOLS, & EQUIPMENT

1. d	2. c	3. b	4. a	5. c
6. b	7. c	8. a	9. b	10. c
11. a	12. c	13. b	14. d	15. c
16. d	17. b	18. a	19. d	20. b
21. c	22. c	23. d	24. a	25. b
26. d	27. c	28. c	29. b	30. a
31. b	32. c	33. b	34. a	35. c
36. d	37. b	38. b	39. c	40. b
41. c	42. a	43. d	44. b	45. c
46. b	47. b	48. a	49. b	50. c

CHAPTER 7: ANATOMY AND PHYSIOLOGY

1. c	2. a	3. d	4. b	5. c
6. b	7. a	8. c	9. a	10. c
11. b	12. d	13. a	14. d	15. b
16. c	17. b	18. d	19. c	20. c
21. d	22. b	23. b	24. b	25. c
26. d	27. a	28. b	29. c	30. c
31. b	32. b	33. c	34. a	35. c
36. c	37. a	38. a	39. b	40. c
41. d	42. a	43. b	44. b	45. c
46. c	47. b	48. d	49. c	50. b
51. b	52. a	53. a	54. d	55. b
56. b	57. c	58. d	59. d	60. c
61. a	62. b	63. d	64. d	65. d
66. c	67. a	68. a	69. b	70. a
71. c	72. a	73. c	74. c	75. a
76. c	77. b	78. d	79. b	80. c
81. a	82. c	83. d	84. c	85. b
86. d	87. c	88. a		

CHAPTER 8: CHEMISTRY

1. d	2. c	3. a	4. a	5. b
6. c	7. b	8. d	9. c	10. c
11. b	12. a	13. c	14. b	15. b
16. a	17. a	18. b	19. c	20. b
21. d	22. a	23. c	24. b	25. a
26. c	27. b	28. d	29. c	30. b
31. c	32. a	33. c	34. b	35. c
36. c	37. a	38. d	39. c	40. b
41. d	42. b	43. d	44. b	45. c
46. a	47. b	48. d	49. b	50. b
51. a	52. a			

CHAPTER 9: ELECTRICITY AND LIGHT THERAPY

1. d	2. a	3. a	4. c
5. b	6. b	7. c	8. d
9. c	10. d	11. b	12. a
13. b	14. b	15. d	16. c
17. a	18. b	19. d	20. a
21. d	22. c	23. c	24. c
25. b	26. a	27. b	28. d
29. c	30. b	31. a	32. a
33. b	34. c	35. b	36. c
37. d	38. d	39. d	40. d

CHAPTER 10: PROPERTIES AND DISORDERS OF THE SKIN

1. c	2. c	3. b	4. a	5. d
6. b	7. c	8. c	9. d	10. b
11. d	12. b	13. b	14. b	15. b
16. c	17. a	18. b	19. b	20. c
21. b	22. d	23. b	24. d	25. b
26. c	27. b	28. a	29. d	30. d
31. c	32. c	33. c	34. c	35. b
36. b	37. a	38. b	39. b	40. c
41. b	42. d	43. d	44. b	45. a
46. b	47. a	48. d	49. a	50. a
51. a	52. d	53. b	54. c	55. c
56. b	57. a	58. c	59. a	60. c
61. a	62. c	63. c	64. b	65. c
66. b	67. c	68. b	69. d	70. a
71. c	72. d	73. b	74. c	75. a
76. b	77. a	78. d	79. a	80. c
81. b	82. c	83. a	84. b	85. c
86. a	87. b	88. c	89. b	90. a

CHAPTER 11: PROPERTIES AND DISORDERS OF THE HAIR AND SCALP

1. b	2. c	3. b	4. c	5. b
6. a	7. c	8. c	9. d	10. d
11. c	12. b	13. b	14. a	15. a
16. b	17. c	18. d	19. b	20. a
21. d	22. b	23. c	24. a	25. c
26. a	27. c	28. d	29. a	30. c
31. b	32. a	33. c	34. a	35. b
36. b	37. a	38. d	39. b	40. d
41. b	42. d	43. b	44. a	45. b
46. c	47. b	48. a	49. b	50. c
51. d	52. b	53. c	54. b	55. c
56. d	57. a	58. b	59. d	60. c
61. d	62. b	63. c	64. a	65. b
66. c	67. a	68. a	69. c	70. a
71. c	72. c	73. d	74. b	75. a
76. b	77. c	78. d	79. b	80. d
81. b	82. a	83. b	84. c	85. b
86. c	87. b	88. d	89. c	90. d
91. c	92. b	93. a	94. d	95. a
96. c	97. c	98.b	99. d	100. b

CHAPTER 12: THE TREATMENT OF HAIR AND SCALP

1. b	2. c	3. b	4. a	5. c
6. b	7. c	8. b	9. a	10. d
11. b	12. a	13. d	14. c	15. b
16. b	17. d	18. a	19. b	20. c
21. b	22. c	23. a	24. b	25. c
26. a	27. d	28. c	29. b	30. c
31. b	32. c	33. d	34. d	35. d
36. b	37. d	38. b	39. c	40. a
41. c	42. a	43. c	44. d	45. c
46. d	47. d	48. d	49. c	50. d
51. d	52. c	53. b	54. c	55. b
56. c	57. b	58. a	59. c	60. d
61. b	62. d	63. c	64. b	65. c
66. b	67. c	68. b	69. a	70. c
71. a	72. b	73. c	74. a	75. c
76. c	77. c	78. d	79. c	80. b

CHAPTER 13: MEN'S FACIAL MASSAGE AND TREATMENTS

1. b	2. d	3. c	4. b	5. d
6. b	7. d	8. c	9. b	10. c
11. c	12. d	13. c	14. a	15. c
16. a	17. b	18. a	19. d	20. d
21. c	22. a	23. c	24. d	25. c
26. b	27. b	28. c	29. d	30. b
31. a	32. c	33. b	34. a	35. a
36. b	37. c	38. a	39. d	40. c
41. b	42. c	43. a	44. c	45. d
46. b	47. a	48. d	49. b	50. c
51. c	52. c	53. d	54. d	55. c
56. b	57. a	58. d	59. b	60. b
61. c	62. b	63. c	64. d	65. c
66. a	67. d	68. c	69. a	70. c
71. a	72. b	73. c	74. d	75. b
76. c	77. d	78. a	79. b	80. b
81. a	82. b	83. d	84. c	85. b
86. b	87. c	88. d	89. c	90. c
91. b	92. a	93. c	94. b	95. c
96. a	97. d	98. c	99. a	100. b

CHAPTER 14: SHAVING AND FACIAL HAIR DESIGN

1. b	2. d	3. b	4. a
5. c	6. b	7. c	8. c
9. b	10. a	11. b	12. b
13. a	14. c	15. b	16. c
17. a	18. b	19. c	20. a
21. c	22. b	23. c	24. d
25. b	26. a	27. c	28. d
29. a	30. c	31. d	32. d
33. a	34. b	35. b	36. d
37. d	38. c	39. a	40. b

CHAPTER 15: MEN'S HAIRCUTTING AND STYLING

1. b	2. a	3. d	4. d	5. b
6. c	7. d	8. c	9. a	10. b
11. d	12. a	13. c	14. b	15. d
16. c	17. a	18. d	19. d	20. b
21. a	22. c	23. a	24. c	25. a
26. d	27. c	28. b	29. a	30. c
31. b	32. c	33. b	34. c	35. a
36. b	37. a	38. c	39. c	40. a
41. b	42. a	43. c	44. a	45. b
46. c	47. b	48. c	49. a	50. c
51. b	52. c	53. d	54. b	55. b
56. d	57. a	58. b	59. c	60. b
61. d	62. a	63. c	64. b	65. d
66. a	67. b	68. c	69. a	70. d
71. c	72. b	73. d	74. b	75. a
76. d	77. b	78. b	79. c	80. b
81. d	82. a	83. c	84. b	85. d
86. b	87. a	88. c	89. a	90. d
91. a	92. d	93. c	94. d	95. c
96. d	97. b	98. c	99. b	100. a

CHAPTER 16: MEN'S HAIRPIECES

1. c	2. b	3. c	4. b	5. a
6. d	7. b	8. c	9. b	10. b
11. a	12. c	13. a	14. c	15. b
16. d	17. c	18. c	19. a	20. b
21. a	22. c	23. b	24. c	25. b
26. a	27. b	28. d	29. b	30. a
31. b	32. c	33. b	34. c	35. d

CHAPTER 17: WOMEN'S HAIRCUTTING AND STYLING

1. c	2. c	3. a	4. b	5. d
6. b	7. c	8. a	9. c	10. d
11. d	12. d	13. b	14. c	15. a
16. b	17. c	18. d	19. a	20. c
21. d	22. a	23. b	24. c	25. b
26. d	27. a	28. a	29. c	30. a
31. b	32. c	33. d	34. a	35. c

CHAPTER 18: CHEMICAL TEXTURE SERVICES

1. b	2. d	3. c	4. a	5. d
6. a	7. c	8. a	9. d	10. b
11. a	12. b	13. d	14. c	15. c
16. a	17. b	18. d	19. b	20. d
21. c	22. a	23. b	24. d	25. c
26. b	27. b	28. c	29. a	30. c
31. b	32. b	33. d	34. a	35. d
36. c	37. d	38. c	39. a	40. c
41. d	42. d	43. b	44. c	45. a
46. b	47. d	48. c	49. a	50. c
51. d	52. d	53. a	54. c	55. b
56. c	57. a	58. d	59. a	60. b
61. c	62. c	63. d	64. b	65. c
66. a	67. d	68. b	69. c	70. a
71. a	72. b	73. d	74. c	75. b
76. a	77. c	78. b	79. a	80. d
81. c	82. d	83. a	84. c	85. b
86. b	87. a	88. d	89. a	90. b
91. c	92. b	93. a	94. b	95. c
96. b	97. b	98. a	99. c	100. b

CHAPTER 19: HAIRCOLORING AND LIGHTENING

1. c	2. a	3. b	4. d	5. a
6. c	7. b	8. b	9. d	10. c
11. b	12. a	13. c	14. a	15. b
16. c	17. d	18. a	19. d	20. b
21. c	22. b	23. c	24. a	25. b
26. b	27. c	28. d	29. a	30. d
31. b	32. c	33. b	34. a	35. a
36. c	37. b	38. d	39. c	40. a
41. d	42. a	43. c	44. c	45. b
46. d	47. a	48. b	49. b	50. d
51. a	52. b	53. c	54. b	55. d
56. d	57. a	58. c	59. b	60. b
61. c	62. a	63. d	64. a	65. c
66. b	67. d	68. c	69. a	70. b
71. d	72. a	73. c	74. b	75. b
76. a	77. b	78. c	79. d	80. a
81. b	82. c	83. b	84. d	85. c
86. a	87. b	88. d	89. b	90. c
91. a	92. b	93. d	94. b	95. a
96. c	97. c	98. a	99. b	100. d

CHAPTER 20: NAILS AND MANICURING

1. c	2. b	3. a	4. b
5. c	6. d	7. b	8. c
9. a	10. a	11. d	12. c
13. a	14. d	15. b	16. c
17. b	18. c	19. d	20. a
21. c	22. a	23. d	24. a
25. c	26. b	27. d	28. a
29. d	30. b	31. d	32. a
33. c	34. b	35. a	36. b
37. c	38. a	39. d	40. a

CHAPTER 21: BARBERSHOP MANAGEMENT

1. d	2. b	3. a	4. c	5. c
6. d	7. b	8. d	9. a	10. b
11. d	12. a	13. c	14. c	15. d
16. b	17. a	18. c	19. b	20. a
21. c	22. b	23. c	24. d	25. d
26. a	27. b	28. d	29. b	30. d
31. a	32. c	33. d	34. c	35. b
36. d	37. a	38. b	39. c	40. a
41. d	42. d	43. c	44. b	45. a

CHAPTER 22: THE JOB SEARCH

1. c	2. d	3. d	4. b
5. d	6. a	7. b	8. d
9. a	10. b	11. a	12. b

CHAPTER 23: STATE BOARD PREPARATION AND LICENSING LAWS

1. c	2. a	3. c	4. d	5. b
6. a	7. b	8. c	9. b	10. d
11. b	12. a	13. c	14. c	15. b
16. d	17. c	18. a	19. c	20. b
21. b	22. d	23. a	24. b	25. d

Answers to Sample State Board Examinations

SAMPLE STATE BOARD EXAMINATION TEST 1

1. b	2. d	3. c	4. d	5. c
6. c	7. b	8. b	9. b	10. d
11. b	12. b	13. b	14. a	15. d
16. d	17. b	18. a	19. c	20. a
21. a	22. c	23. d	24. d	25. c
26. c	27. b	28. c	29. d	30. b
31. c	32. c	33. a	34. b	35. a
36. b	37. d	38. c	39. a	40. b
41. a	42. c	43. b	44. b	45. d
46. b	47. a	48. d	49. c	50. d
51. b	52. a	53. c	54. d	55. c
56. b	57. c	58. a	59. a	60. d
61. b	62. a	63. d	64. b	65. a
66. c	67. a	68. c	69. c	70. d
71. a	72. d	73. d	74. b	75. c
76. d	77. b	78. c	79. c	80. b
81. b	82. d	83. a	84. c	85. d
86. c	87. b	88. a	89. b	90. c
91. c	92. a	93. a	94. c	95. a
96. c	97. d	98. b	99. a	100. b
101. a	102. c	103. d	104. c	105. b
106. c	107. c	108. b	109. c	110. a
111. b	112. b	113. c	114. d	115. b
116. a	117. c	118. d	119. b	120. d
121. a	122. b	123. a	124. d	125. b
126. b	127. b	128. a	129. a	130. d
131. a	132. d	133. d	134. b	135. b
136. b	137. c	138. b	139. b	140. c
141. a	142. a	143. d	144. b	145. a
146. d	147. c	148. b	149. b	150. a

SAMPLE STATE BOARD EXAMINATION TEST 2

1. b	2. d	3. d	4. c	5. b
6. b	7. a	8. b	9. c	10. d
11. b	12. a	13. b	14. a	15. d
16. d	17. b	18. a	19. c	20. a
21. a	22. c	23. d	24. d	25. c
26. c	27. b	28. c	29. d	30. b
31. c	32. c	33. a	34. d	35. a
36. c	37. d	38. d	39. a	40. b
41. a	42. c	43. b	44. c	45. d
46. b	47. b	48. d	49. b	50. d
51. b	52. a	53. d	54. d	55. c
56. b	57. c	58. b	59. a	60. d
61. b	62. a	63. d	64. b	65. a
66. c	67. a	68. c	69. c	70. d
71. a	72. d	73. d	74. c	75. b
76. d	77. b	78. c	79. c	80. b
81. b	82. d	83. a	84. c	85. d
86. a	87. b	88. a	89. b	90. c
91. c	92. c	93. a	94. a	95. a
96. c	97. c	98. b	99. a	100. b
101. a	102. c	103. d	104. c	105. b
106. c	107. c	108. b	109. a	110. d
111. c	112. c	113. a	114. d	115. b
116. a	117. c	118. d	119. d	120. a
121. a	122. b	123. a	124. d	125. b
126. b	127. a	128. b	129. c	130. d
131. a	132. d	133. d	134. b	135. a
136. b	137. c	138. b	139. b	140. c
141. a	142. a	143. d	144. b	145. a
146. d	147. c	148. b	149. a	150. a

SAMPLE STATE BOARD EXAMINATION TEST 3

1. a	2. d	3. d	4. c	5. b
6. b	7. a	8. b	9. a	10. d
11. b	12. a	13. b	14. a	15. d
16. d	17. b	18. a	19. c	20. a
21. a	22. c	23. d	24. d	25. c
26. c	27. b	28. c	29. d	30. b
31. c	32. c	33. a	34. d	35. a
36. c	37. d	38. d	39. a	40. b
41. a	42. c	43. d	44. c	45. d
46. b	47. b	48. d	49. b	50. d
51. b	52. a	53. d	54. d	55. c
56. b	57. c	58. b	59. a	60. d
61. b	62. a	63. d	64. b	65. a
66. c	67. a	68. c	69. c	70. d
71. a	72. d	73. d	74. c	75. c
76. d	77. b	78. c	79. c	80. b
81. b	82. d	83. a	84. c	85. d
86. a	87. b	88. c	89. b	90. c
91. c	92. c	93. a	94. a	95. a
96. c	97. c	98. b	99. a	100. b
101. a	102. c	103. d	104. c	105. b
106. c	107. c	108. b	109. a	110. d
111. c	112. c	113. a	114. d	115. b
116. a	117. c	118. d	119. d	120. a
121. a	122. c	123. b	124. d	125. b
126. b	127. a	128. b	129. c	130. d
131. a	132. d	133. d	134. b	135. a
136. b	137. c	138. b	139. b	140. c
141. a	142. a	143. d	144. b	145. a
146. d	147. c	148. b	149. a	150. a

Part III: Helpful Reminders for Examination Day

The following reminders have been prepared for your benefit and will assist you in passing the state board examinations.

1. *Take the time to present a professional appearance.* This includes your clothing, personal hygiene, general health, and posture.

2. *Adopt a positive mental attitude.* Doing so will help you to overcome the nervousness often associated with taking test and exams. It might help to remember that state board exams are not given to make candidates fail, but to do justice to all candidates using measurable and objective methods of evaluation. Testing and evaluation are vital to determining a candidate's competency for the profession.

3. *Be prepared.* Create a checklist of the supplies and tools you will need for both exams. Be guided by the candidate information that usually accompanies confirmation of the test date. Make sure you bring a photo ID for identification purposes.

4. *Be punctual.* Learn in advance how to reach the test site and allow sufficient time for travel. Being on time for the exam will alleviate some stress and make it easier to maintain a positive attitude so that you can do your best.

5. *Written or computer-based tests.* Some general reminders for written or computer-based testing include the following:
   - Be ready to begin when the signal is given by the test proctor.
   - Scan the entire test before beginning to answer the questions. Then, read each test item carefully and answer the questions consecutively whenever possible.
   - Avoid spending too much time on one test item; if in doubt, continue with the test and return to the unanswered item(s) after completing the entire test.
   - If time permits, review all your answers before submitting the completed test.

6. *Practical exams.* General reminders for practical exams include:
   - Ask questions of the examiner before the signal to begin is given. Talking is prohibited during the exam.
   - Observe all sanitation rules during the practical exam. The use of proper sanitation methods is vital to a passing score.
   - Use only clean and sanitized tools and implements.
   - Wash your hands before beginning each service.
   - Make sure your model is draped correctly for each service.
   - Do not put combs or implements in pockets.
   - Do not set a tool or implement down and reuse it without sanitizing it first.